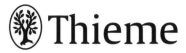

# Encyclopedia of Football Medicine

## Volume 3: Protecting the Player

**Tim Meyer, MD, PhD**
Head of the Institute of Sports and
  Preventive Medicine
Saarland University
Team Doctor
German National Team
Chair of Medical Committee
German Football Association

**Ian Beasley, MD**
Former Head of Medical Services
English Football Association
Doctor
Senior Men's Team
London, England

**Zoran Bahtijarevic, MD**
National Team Doctor
Croatian Football Team
CEO of Children's Hospital
Zagreb, Croatia

**Grégory Dupont, PhD**
Head of Performance
Lille FC (LOSC)
Associate Researcher,
University of Lille
Lille, France

**Mike Earl**
Former UEFA Medical and Anti-Doping
  Manager
Switzerland
World Rugby Anti-Doping General Manager,
Dublin, Ireland

**Jan Ekstrand, MD, PhD**
Professor of Sports Medicine and Orthopaedic
  Surgeon
Football Research Group & Division of Community
  Medicine
Department of Medical and Health Sciences
Linköping University, Sweden

**Ronald J. Maughan, PhD**
Visiting Professor
School of Medicine
St Andrews University
St. Andrews, Scotland

**Jason Palmer**
Head of Physiotherapy
Chelsea Football Club,
London, England

**Christopher Willis, PhD**
Lead Expert of Performance Coaching for Special
  Forces and High Performance Athletes
CEO of Centre of Mental Excellence Gmbh
Innsbruck, Austria

67 illustrations

Thieme
Stuttgart • New York • Delhi • Rio de Janeiro

Library of Congress Cataloging-in-Publication Data is available from the publisher.

© 2017 by Georg Thieme Verlag KG

Thieme Publishers Stuttgart
Rüdigerstrasse 14, 70469 Stuttgart, Germany
+49 [0]711 8931 421, customerservice@thieme.de

Thieme Publishers New York
333 Seventh Avenue, New York, NY 10001 USA
+1 800 782 3488, customerservice@thieme.com

Thieme Publishers Delhi
A-12, Second Floor, Sector-2, Noida-201301
Uttar Pradesh, India
+91 120 45 566 00, customerservice@thieme.in

Thieme Publishers Rio, Thieme Publicações Ltda.
Edifício Rodolpho de Paoli, 25º andar
Av. Nilo Peçanha, 50 – Sala 2508
Rio de Janeiro 20020-906 Brasil
+55 21 3172 2297 / +55 21 3172 1896

Cover design: Thieme Publishing Group
Photographs – Getty Images, UEFA
(All football images including the cover.)
Typesetting by Ditech Process Solutions, India

Printed in India by Replika Press Pvt. Ltd.    5 4 3 2 1

ISBN 978-3-13-240872-2

Also available as an e-book:
eISBN 978-3-13-220371-6

**Important note:** Medicine is an ever-changing science undergoing continual development. Research and clinical experience are continually expanding our knowledge, in particular our knowledge of proper treatment and drug therapy. Insofar as this book mentions any dosage or application, readers may rest assured that the authors, editors, and publishers have made every effort to ensure that such references are in accordance with **the state of knowledge at the time of production of the book.**

Nevertheless, this does not involve, imply, or express any guarantee or responsibility on the part of the publishers in respect to any dosage instructions and forms of applications stated in the book. **Every user is requested to examine carefully** the manufacturers' leaflets accompanying each drug and to check, if necessary in consultation with a physician or specialist, whether the dosage schedules mentioned therein or the contraindications stated by the manufacturers differ from the statements made in the present book. Such examination is particularly important with drugs that are either rarely used or have been newly released on the market. Every dosage schedule or every form of application used is entirely at the user's own risk and responsibility. The authors and publishers request every user to report to the publishers any discrepancies or inaccuracies noticed. If errors in this work are found after publication, errata will be posted at www.thieme.com on the product description page.

Some of the product names, patents, and registered designs referred to in this book are in fact registered trademarks or proprietary names even though specific reference to this fact is not always made in the text. Therefore, the appearance of a name without designation as proprietary is not to be construed as a representation by the publisher that it is in the public domain.

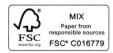

# Contents

# Foreword

As modern football has progressed in recent years, the role of the team doctor has become ever more important to the success of its teams, not only in protecting the health and fitness of players, but also in providing a comprehensive and scientifically advanced medical support service. The role of the doctor now encompasses medical team planning and management, first aid techniques, injury prevention, health promotion, rehabilitation, and many more areas, meaning that the doctor is now one of the key positions in any successful football team.

As an organization, UEFA always seeks to further scientific research and to provide the best standards of medical care for players, and these books bring together some of the most eminent practitioners in all aspects of the now very specific domain of football medicine. All areas of the modern football doctor's toolkit are covered with advice on advanced treatment techniques, management of the medical team, and best practice in all areas of the doctor's role. UEFA's many years of work in football medicine and the extensive experience of the chapter authors make this an indispensable text for any doctor wishing to work in the field.

As we look toward the future and the further development and dissemination of football-specific medical expertise, I hope that this book will serve you well as a reference guide in a sport that is now so technically and scientifically advanced to be almost unrecognizable from the one within which I started my career.

I hope that you will enjoy this book and the book series.

*Michel D'Hooghe, MD*
*Bruges, Belgium*

# Preface

The third and last volume of the *Encyclopedia of Football Medicine*, entitled *Health and Performance*, is concerned with the health of football players at all levels of the game. The content of this third volume was initially developed as the course manual of the third and last workshop of the UEFA Football Doctor Education Programme, which took place in Budapest in 2015. The book explores the various issues that can affect the player's health and well-being, each developed by experts in the specific field.

Prof. Tim Meyer, the German Football Association (DFB) team doctor, and Prof. Ian Beasley, the former English Football Association (FA) team doctor, were contracted as the course leaders of this workshop and took the lead in the development of the program. The team doctor is expected to be an expert in many different and highly specialized areas that may influence injury, health, and well-being of players: these are additional to the fundamental issues covered in Volumes 1 and 2. Staying abreast of the ever-expanding literature in all of these areas is a major challenge, and the team doctor must inevitably rely on experts to assist with the analysis and interpretation of this evidence. The two course leaders therefore recruited six other authors, recognized as international experts in their area of expertise.

UEFA Medical Committee Vice-Chairman and UEFA Injury Study leader, Prof. Jan Ekstrand, introduced the book with a chapter on injury prevention that includes his findings that traditional injury prevention methods may not be sufficient at elite level. This chapter is followed by a review of the evidence on rehabilitation in football medicine, written by Jason Palmer, the Head of Physiotherapy and Therapy Services at Chelsea FC. The third chapter is written by Sport Psychologist Chris Willis, who focuses on general mental health and psychological issues relating to football, and the key instruments of a toolkit for the modern football doctor. Prof. Ronald J. Maughan, Expert in Sport and Exercise Nutrition at St Andrews University, reviews the role of nutrition and dietary supplements in maintaining health and performance and in promoting recovery. The book then moves on to the monitoring of fatigue and recovery in football, with a review from Grégory Dupont, Head of Sports Science at LOSC Lille. The book further covers UEFA's principal fight against doping by instructing the team doctors on their main responsibilities in this regard. UEFA Doping Control Officer and team doctor of the Croatian National Football Team, Dr. Zoran Bahtijarevic, and former UEFA Medical and Anti-Doping manager, Mike Earl, developed this chapter to be an essential guide to team doctors. In Chapter 8, Prof. Ian Beasley advises team doctors on how to prepare best for away matches (particularly when travelling overseas) and final tournaments. The book ends with Prof. Tim Meyer reviewing the different considerations in the screening of players for elite football, both for pre-competition fitness/eligibility and for pre-transfer signings.

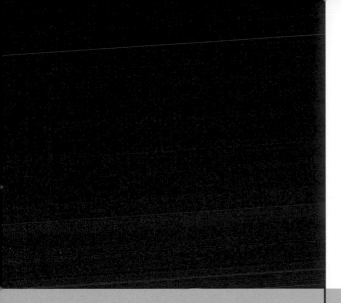

# Chapter 1

## Injury Prevention

*Jan Ekstrand*

The aim of this chapter is to describe how to prevent injuries in elite-level football and how to "keep the players on the pitch." As has been shown by the results of the Union of European Football Association (UEFA) Elite Club Injury Study (ECIS), clubs who have more of their players available during the season will be likely to be more successful, and as such, injury prevention has become a key contributor to the success of a modern football team.

## 1.1  Why Injury Prevention?

The protection of players is a key responsibility for all involved in football, certainly from an ethical perspective. However, it is particularly important for the medical team. Besides the humanitarian aspects of protecting the players from short- and long-term injury and their associated consequences, there are important performance and economic reasons to try to avoid injuries and keep players on the pitch.

The risk of injury for athletes participating in professional football is substantial. It has been estimated that the overall risk is about 1,000 times higher than for typical industrial occupations generally regarded as high risk.[1] As reported by Ekstrand et al,[2] the impact of injuries on team performance can be considerable when, on average, 14% of the squad are unavailable due to injury at any point during the season. As shown in the UEFA ECIS,[3] injuries have a significant influence on performance in both national and European competitions in male professional football. In addition, injuries also carry an economic cost. Recently, it was reported that the average cost for a first team UEFA Champions League (UCL) player injured for 1 month is around 600,000.00 Euros.[4] The findings of the study clearly show how injury prevention can increase a team's chances of success.

## 1.2  Is It Possible to Prevent Injuries?

As early as 1983, Ekstrand et al[5] published the results of the first injury prevention trials in football. The authors evaluated an injury prevention program in a randomized trial at male amateur level. The seven-part program included (1) the correction of training, (2) provision of optimum equipment, (3) prophylactic ankle taping in players with clinical instability or history of previous strain, (4) controlled rehabilitation, (5) exclusion of players with serious knee instability, (6) information about the importance of disciplined play and the increased risk of injury at training camps, and (7) correction and supervision by physicians and physical therapists. The intervention and the control teams were followed up after 6 months. The rate of injury was 75% lower in the intervention teams than in the control teams (**Fig. 1.1**).

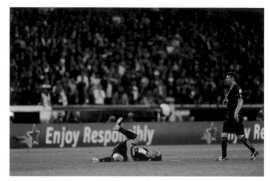

**Fig. 1.1**  There are important performance and economic reasons to try to avoid injuries and keep players on the pitch.

## 1.3  A Model of Prevention

It is well described how injuries can be prevented theoretically. A four-step model for injury prevention has been outlined by van Mechelen and this model has been widely used to implement preventive measures in sports.[6] However, recently other different models have been proposed, which include the addition of two further steps to van Mechelen's model. These two new steps are referred to as "implementation" and "compliance," and are considered necessary in order to make prevention more effective in "real-life situations."[7,8,9,10] They are especially important in order to achieve a positive effect in elite-level clubs (**Fig. 1.2**).

The different steps are described below.

**STEP 1: ESTABLISH THE EXTENT OF THE INJURY PROBLEM—INJURY STATISTICS**

Analysis of the injury problem by identifying and describing the incidence, the severity, and the pattern of injuries is the first step in preventing injuries. Elite clubs participating in the UEFA ECIS receive such information each season. This study design follows the consensus statement reached by Fédération Internationale de Football Association (FIFA) and UEFA on how to carry out injury studies and receive reliable statistical information.[11,12] The advantage of participation is that clubs can compare their own data with data from other clubs or other groups using the same study design. They can then find out in which areas their injury situation is favorable or in line with other clubs, and (more importantly) it can help the medical team evaluate problem areas. Teams not participating in the ECIS can also use the same method of data collection and then evaluate their own injury situation by comparing with results published from the UEFA study. Forms and manuals for the UEFA study can be received from the UEFA Medical Unit. Often clubs and/or national teams will have their own internal statistics models, which may be effective, but which cannot allow comparison of results with other teams.

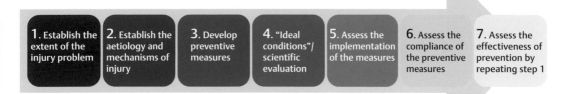

1. Establish the extent of the injury problem

2. Establish the aetiology and mechanisms of injury

3. Develop preventive measures

4. "Ideal conditions"/ scientific evaluation

5. Assess the implementation of the measures

6. Assess the compliance of the preventive measures

7. Assess the effectiveness of prevention by repeating step 1

**Fig. 1.2** Sequence of prevention of football injuries. (Adapted from van Mechelen et al 1992,[6] Finch 2006,[7] and Verhagen 2014.[9])

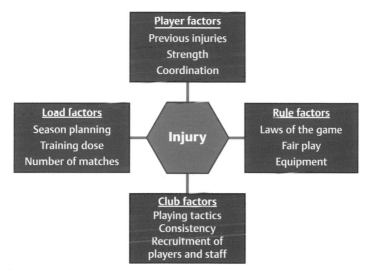

**Player factors**
Previous injuries
Strength
Coordination

**Load factors**
Season planning
Training dose
Number of matches

**Injury**

**Rule factors**
Laws of the game
Fair play
Equipment

**Club factors**
Playing tactics
Consistency
Recruitment of
players and staff

**Fig. 1.3** Risk factors for injury.

STEP 2: ESTABLISH THE ETIOLOGY AND MECHANISMS OF INJURY

The second step is to identify the risk factors and mechanisms behind injuries. Knowledge of risk factors and injury mechanisms is necessary in order to work out effective preventive measures against injuries. The causes of football injuries are often multifactorial and there are usually a number of risk factors involved. Examples of risk factors that could contribute to injuries are shown in **Fig. 1.3**.

## 1.4 Evaluating Risk Factors

Risk factors can be divided in four major categories:
- Player factors.
- Load factors.
- Club factors.
- Rule factors.

## 1.4.1 Player Factors (Intrinsic Factors)

**NOTE:**
These factors can be physical or psychological.

The findings concerning the relationship between age and injury in adult male elite players are contradictory. Arnason et al[13] found increasing age to be a significant risk factor for injuries in general; the odds ratio was 1.1 per year. This finding has been verified in the UEFA ECIS.[14] However, different injury types seem to have different associations with injury risk. Muscle injury in general has been reported to increase with age.[13] However, when separated into different muscle groups, as in the UEFA study, an increased incidence with age was found only for calf muscle injuries and not for hamstring, quadriceps, or hip/groin strains.[15,16] Older players (above 30 years) had a sixfold increased rate of calf injury compared to players under 21 years of age and an almost twofold increased rate compared to players between 22 and 30 years.[16]

The theory behind the increase of injury risk with age is that increasing age leads to less elasticity and strength in tissues, which means that they can withstand less load and are more easily damaged. However, the age span at elite level is quite narrow (18–35 years), and it is doubtful whether strength and tissue elasticity vary within it. The UEFA ECIS revealed an increased risk of injury with age but with a peak rate among players aged 29 to 30 years.[14] Also, as pointed out by Kristenson et al,[14] older players who are still able to compete at elite level may be less injury prone than players who retired early from professional football. Thus, selection of less injury-prone players who managed to stay in the UEFA elite cohort may have contributed to the lack of increase in injury risk also involving the oldest players.

In contrast, other types of injuries, such as overuse injuries, are more common in younger players. Players in the UEFA study who sustained stress fractures were significantly younger than those that did not.[17] The change of load when moving from an academy environment or a lower level of play might be an explanation for this finding.[17]

**Previous injury** is an important risk factor for new injuries.[13,18] An elite-level player injured during one season has a threefold increased risk of suffering any kind of new injury during the following season; hence the more injuries a player sustains during a season, the higher the risk in the following season.[18] The recurrence rate of football injuries could reflect insufficient rehabilitation. In the UEFA ECIS, a reinjury is defined as an injury of the same type and at the same location as an index injury occurring within 2 months after return to full participation from the index injury. The total reinjury rate is around 16%,[2] but substantially higher (18–29%) for overuse injuries.[17,19,20]

A further finding from the UEFA study is that players at the early stages of their careers in elite football (19 years) had a lower general injury rate than more established players (26 years) but a higher rate of stress-related bone injuries.[14]

**Anthropometric factors** (such as height, weight, body composition, percentage of fat or body mass index [BMI]) have not been found as risk factors for injuries at male elite level.[16,18,21]

A popular claim is that **muscle strength** is correlated to injury risk, especially to muscle injuries. However, this is a claim that has been difficult to substantiate in scientific studies due to inadequacies in the ability to measure muscle strength.[22] Frequently, muscle strength is measured using isokinetic measuring apparatus. The reliability of such measurements is high, with very similar results achieved in repeated measurements. However, the validity is low, as sitting strapped in a chair and moving the leg slowly is far from replicating football activity.

The same problem is faced when measuring *coordination*. This is usually done in a laboratory testing environment with the player standing on one leg on the floor or on a force platform. Again, any resemblance with movements on a football field is very low.

In a multivariate study of risk factors for football injuries, Arnason et al[13] found that previous injury and age were the physical risk factors identified, whereas no other fitness variables measured (height, weight, body composition, flexibility, leg strength, jumping ability, aerobic capacity, and joint stability) could predict injury.

**Psychological factors** such as personality, goals, motivation, self-confidence, ability to withstand stress, and susceptibility to risk determine a player's performance in footballing situations. Psychological training is sometimes used to try and improve the performance of individual players or the whole team; however, the connection between psychological factors and risk of injury is seldom discussed and the area has been subject to little scientific study.

### 1.4.2 Load Factors (Extrinsic Factors)

**NOTE:**

Load on players is an important extrinsic factor. Overloading could be physical or psychological.

Factors like content, intensity, and duration of training as well as numbers of, and intervals between, matches and restitution between training and matches are important to avoid physical and psychological fatigue in players.

A congested football calendar can negatively affect the well-being of players. Studies have shown that it takes several days to fully recover following a football match. Remaining fatigue up until 72 hours after a football match has been shown in terms of decreased physical performance, as well as through increased levels of blood markers indicating muscle damage and oxidative stress.[23,24] In addition, psychological preparation and travels before a match may further contribute to fatigue.[25] Playing professional football matches, especially when playing away, is associated with long travels and unfamiliar sleeping environments which may have a negative impact on the quality of sleep for the players.[26] These factors are discussed in more detail in Chapter 5.

The correlation between match exposure of European footballers before the World Cup 2002 and their injuries and performances during that World Cup has been studied.[25] There is a considerable variation in the number of matches played per season in European professional leagues, and top-level players are obliged to play many matches, especially during the final period of the season. This study indicates that a period with a congested match calendar can lead to fatigue, increasing the risk of injury, and poor performance during the following period.

Dellal et al[27] reported similar results, where a congested calendar (six consecutive matches, each separated by 3 days) increased match injury rates and Dupont et al[28] found a five times increased injury risk in matches with 4 or less days' recovery compared with matches with 6 or more days' recovery. Recently, Bengtsson et al[29] reported that match congestion was associated with increased muscle injury rates but had no, or very limited, influence on team performance.

The balance between training and matches might also influence the injury rates. Ekstrand et al,[30] studying the relation between training and matches at amateur levels, found that a high training/match quotient with many training sessions in relation to the number of matches played gave greater success and fewer injuries. However, this relation has not been studied at the professional level.

**Measurement of load on training and matches.** The ability to measure load on football players is a topic of great interest for evaluating mechanisms behind injuries. The ultimate objective of load measurements is to be able to evaluate the effect of strategies to reduce the risk of injuries for football players by regulation of match play and training participation. In professional clubs, different systems are used for evaluating load on players; Global Positioning System (GPS) measurement is most commonly used. This enables the measurement of player position, distance travelled, velocity, and movement patterns. However, there is currently no consensus on which type of measurement instruments to use and which variables to collect, and no data available on GPS variables have so far been correlated to injuries. GPS measurements are mainly used for performance purposes and so far there is no evidence of their value in predicting injuries. Some clubs claim that GPS measurement of load is of value in the rehabilitation process after injury, but scientific evidence is still lacking. Other methods for evaluating load are to measure heart rate variability, Borg rating of perceived exertion (RPE) scale or Profile of Mood States (POMS) tests; however, none of these have so far been scientifically proven to predict injuries.

## 1.4.3 Club Factors (Extrinsic Factors)

**NOTE:**
These factors are scarcely studied, but may be more important at the elite level than previously understood.

**Playing tactics** is a factor to consider. It is well known that the risk of injury is highest on matches (the higher the more important the matches are).[22] Furthermore, the majority (around 70–80%) of match injuries occur in contact situations. Teams and players with a very technical playing style (one-touch passes, etc.) have less contact situations and less risk of contact injuries.

**Internal communication** within the team seems to be a very important factor for keeping the players on the pitch. According to the majority of doctors and physical therapists participating in the UEFA ECIS, this factor is the single most important factor for avoiding injuries, and analyses from the study seems to verify such opinions.

**Club consistency** is another factor to consider. A change within the technical staff behind the team is common between seasons (new head coaches often bring their own technical staff to the new club), but it also occurs during a season (change of head coach due to negative results is commonly seen). New coaching staff frequently introduce changes (in training methods and load, for example). Changes might have a negative effect on the injury risk since the human body does not tolerate quick changes of load. It takes time for the connective tissue to adapt and it is well known that too rapid increase of load or change of load increases the risk of overuse injuries especially.

**Recruitment of players** and staff is also a factor to consider. It is well known that players with previous injuries are at a higher risk of sustaining new injuries.[18] The selection of the team and the signing of new players are important, and in some ways predict the injury situation for the upcoming season (as, e.g., signing a player with a previous injury record could be anticipated to increase the club's overall injury rate due to their increased risk of reinjury). Furthermore, the selection of a coach is important both for performance and injury risk, since data from the UEFA ECIS show that coaches with consistently low injury rates (in the same or in different clubs) win more trophies, as they play more matches with their strongest team.

**Human and financial resources** for medical teams could be a factor as this varies between teams at elite level. Some clubs have one or several full-time team doctors, while other team doctors work only part

1

time. Furthermore, some teams have physical therapists acting as personal trainers (two to three players
per physical therapist with the aim of creating a
closer contact with players); other teams have a few
physical therapists working for the whole squad. No
single configuration of human resources and staff
specialisms can be considered an optimal model (as
each team will vary in its needs); nor can it be
assumed that greater financial resources for a medical unit will automatically produce better results on
injury management. However, limiting resources
where a clear need exists could provide a false economy for the team if this leads to high-value players
incurring time loss from injuries that could have
been prevented through better resource allocation.

### 1.4.4  Rule Factors (Extrinsic Factors)

The **Laws of the Game** are decided by the International Football Association Board (IFAB) and are published by FIFA. In recent years, rules have been
changed with the aim of improving injury prevention. Details about the medical aspects of the Laws of
the Game can be found in Chapter 2 of the FDEP
Workshop 2 manual.

It is reasonable to suggest that although the behavior
of players is key, a *referee* may influence the risk of
injury by the way he or she interprets the regulations. *Foul play* (according to the decisions of the referee) is involved in around 25 to 30% of all match
injuries, the majority being due to opponent fouls;
hence, where foul play can be reduced or discouraged, it can be assumed that this will help to reduce
injury risk.[31]

The use of **equipment** is outlined in the Laws of the
Game. *Shin guards* are intended for protection of the
lower leg and the use of shin guards is obligatory in
all football matches.

The correlation between *boots* and injuries has not
been evaluated in football due to the complexity of
accurate measurement. For such a study to take
place, this would require measurement of the exposure for different boots and boot types. However, as
elite players will use many different boots and sometimes have modifications (putting extra studs, etc.),
producing meaningful results would be difficult.

The **shoe–surface connection** is also important but
rarely studied.[32] A good grip (high friction) between
boot and the ground creates large twisting forces in
the knee; however, a good grip is necessary for the
player to change direction rapidly.[22] Friction
between foot and ground should be within an optimal range; too much friction increases the risk of
injury and too little friction decreases the performance of the player.[32]

Recent studies have shown a difference in injury risk
and injury pattern in different **geographical regions**
with different climates.[33,34] Teams from regions with
a cooler climate had a higher injury incidence in general compared to teams with a warmer climate, possibly due to the effect of a cooler climate on pitches.
However, the anterior cruciate ligament (ACL) injury
incidence followed the reverse trend and was higher
in teams with a warmer climate. The higher ACL
injury risk associated with warmer climates could be
due to an increased shoe–surface traction.

### 1.4.5  Who Is in Control of Injury Risk Factors?

Only those with influence over risk factors are able
to modify them. **Fig. 1.4** illustrates a simplified
model of injury risk factors. The medical team has a
close contact with the players and can normally provide players with different individual training programs and other individual preventive measures
influencing player factors. Load on players is normally decided by the coaching staff, while team factors are mainly influenced by the CEO, the board,
and the President of the club, or the General Secre-
tary of the National Association.

**STEP 3: DEVELOP PREVENTIVE METHODS**

The third step is to develop preventive methods based
on the information gained from steps 1 and 2. There
are many suggestions of how to prevent football injuries but few controlled trials. The few trials showing a
positive effect of preventive measures on the total
injury incidence have all used a multimodal approach
by including a program of different preventive measures[5,35,36] including player factors, load factors (adaptation of training, education of coaches), rules (fair
play), and equipment factors. Other studies have
shown a positive effect of preventive actions aiming to
reduce specific injuries such as ankle sprains[37] or hamstring muscle injuries.[38]

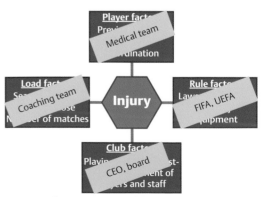

**Fig. 1.4**  Influences on injury risk factors.

### 1.4.6 Methods Designed to Address Player Factors

The following are preventive methods frequently used at elite-level clubs.

### Strength Training

The assumption that strength training is valuable for the prevention of injuries has been difficult to substantiate in scientific studies. One reason could be that there are still difficulties in measuring muscle strength. Muscle strength is usually measured using isokinetic measuring apparatus (see **Fig. 1.5**). The reliability of isokinetic measurements of thigh muscle strength is high (the measurement error being small), and the same results can be achieved after repeated measurements, and if collected by different testers. However, the validity is low, as the measurements do not accurately mimic football movements. Measurement in a laboratory setting takes place at movement speeds of between 30 and 300 degrees per second. However, in rapid football actions like shooting, the movement speed of the shooting leg has been estimated to be around 900 degrees per second. Furthermore, in a laboratory setting, the player is strapped to a chair, which differs significantly from the body position a player would adopt on the football field.

It has been claimed that an imbalance in muscle strength, for example, between right and left would increase the risk of injury, but these measurements are not universally accepted. When measuring the HQ quotient, that is, the quotient of muscle strength between the hamstrings (H) and the quadriceps (Q), problems arise in the measurement technique. If one measures the quotient between peak torque for the quadriceps and hamstrings, the peaks are at different angles for the knee.[22]

It is quite possible that muscle strength in the thigh is important in protecting against injury to the knee, but the available measurement methods are insufficient to demonstrate this.

### Stretching and Flexibility Training

Stretching and flexibility training is commonly used in football. Stretching has been included in preventive programs,[5] but has never been tested as an isolated measure to prevent injuries. The reason for this could well be that stretching is so commonly used that it is difficult to find a control group not using stretching. The fact that there are no scientific studies backing up the use of a method does not necessarily exclude the possibility that it is effective.

### Co-Ordination

Co-ordination is the ability to activate the muscular system and to coordinate movements, and is important in all football activities. There is much clinical evidence to suggest that training co-ordination is an important factor in preventing many types of injuries. However, the scientific evidence is sparse, probably because of difficulties in measuring co-ordination. The commonly used methods of evaluating co-ordination are stabilometry measurements and Solec (standing on one leg eyes closed); however, both have inherent problems with reliability and validity as standing still on one leg is hardly a football-specific activity. However, ankle disk training has been shown to be effective in the prevention of ankle and knee ligament injuries.[37,39]

### Ankle Taping

Preventative taping of a previously injured ankle reduces the risk of the injury recurring.[37] There are, however, no studies that have shown that taping a healthy ankle is beneficial. There are various theories concerning why taping the ankle acts as an injury prophylaxis. One theory is that a tape bandage gives rise to a mechanical improvement in ankle stability. It has been shown, however, that the tape gradually loosens during physical activity, while still restricting the ankle's movement outward. Another theory is that the tape bandage irritates the skin, causing a reflex in which the muscles surrounding the ankle tighten, which has a stabilizing effect.

### Aerobic Capacity

At elite level, the incidence of match injuries has increasing tendency over time in both the first and the second halves.[31] One might speculate that fatigue might be an explanation for these findings. Studies

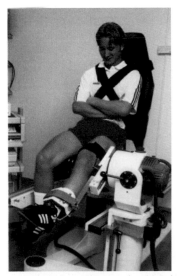

**Fig. 1.5** Measuring thigh muscle strength using isokinetic apparatus.

**1**

of physical demands in football have shown that fatigue develops toward the end of a game, and consequently the amount of high-intensity running and technical performance is lowered. The aerobic capacity of the player is a factor that may influence the player's risk of sustaining an injury. In a study at amateur level, the incidence of ligament injuries tended to be lower in players with higher aerobic capacity,[40] but no study at the elite level has so far been reported.

### Psychological Training

Psychology, behavior, and well-being have all been suggested to be important factors in contributing to the risk of injuries. A recent study indicated that trait anxiety, negative-life-event stress, and daily issues were significant predictors of injury among professional football players.[41] This area is covered in more detail in Chapter 3.

### Preseason Examination

The UEFA club licensing system (which is also valid in most national associations) states: "The licence applicant must ensure that all its players eligible to play for its first squad undergo a yearly medical examination, including a cardiovascular screening. The club's doctor is solely responsible that the requested players' medical examination has been duly performed." So, carrying out a yearly medical examination of the players is mandatory at elite level.

A preseason check-up is an ideal opportunity for the medical team to get to know the players, to establish a good contact with them, and to evaluate their general health including previous injuries and possible remaining sequels after previous injuries. The examination will also provide an idea of the player's normal level of mobility in the joints and any instability can be noted from previous injuries. If new injuries should occur during the season, it is important to be aware of the condition of the joint before the injury.

A preseason examination is also a good opportunity to analyze and correct individual factors that could trigger injuries. If such weaknesses are eliminated by means of injury prevention methods, the risk of injury during the season can be reduced. This concept is mostly valid for players with previous injuries with remaining weaknesses.[13] For previously uninjured players, so far it has not been shown that either preseason screening can predict injuries later during the season or preventive measures based on screening results are effective.

A screening can also be valuable from a psychological point of view as it provides a sense of security for the player, if he/she believes that the club is doing everything it can to minimize the risk of injuries.

Precompetition medical screening is considered in more detail in Chapter 9.

### Rehabilitation, Avoiding Reinjuries

Since reinjuries are so common in football, strategies to reduce their occurrence can be a very important preventive measure. In the UEFA ECIS, the reinjury rates differ substantially between clubs (between 5 and 25%). the definitions in the UEFA study state that "a player with an injury is considered injured until the medical team gives an ok for full participation in training and matches." This means that a reinjury within 2 months could be considered as a failure of the medical team. However, in real life it is more complicated. Sometimes the advice from the medical team might be overruled by the coaching team or the players, and sometimes calculated risks are taken in important matches. However, putting safety concerns above pressures to return the player too quickly could be a way of reducing the reinjury rate (**Fig. 1.6**).

The main problem is in accurately evaluating when a player is ready to return to training and matches. There is so far a lack of consensus on how to objectively conduct such an evaluation. Many tests to date have lacked either validity (by being not sufficiently football specific) or reliability.

### 1.4.7 Methods Designed to Address Load Factors

The load on players should be within an optimal range; too little load is negative from the performance perspective, and too much load increases the risk of injury. Overloading could be physical or psychological and could be short term (e.g., overload from specific training sessions with new training regimes or fatigue from long matches) or long term (e.g., too many matches during a long season).

The key to avoid overloading is to monitor the players. The purpose of monitoring is to control the

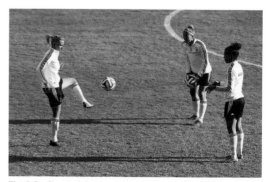

**Fig. 1.6** Since reinjuries are so common in football, strategies to reduce their occurrence can be a very important preventive measure.

prescribed stimulus and avoid overtraining, overuse, and chronic fatigue. *Personal monitoring* of players carried out by the team technical staff is probably the most effective way to avoid physical and psychological overload. The human body uses pain as a warning system for physical overload; however, players can also show signs of psychological overload or burnout. Early symptoms can include sleep disturbances, anger, irritation, and lack of motivation.

A player must listen to their body and learn where his/her training threshold is. The technical staff (coaches and medical team) must also watch for signs of overexertion in players. In connection with this, it is important for the coach to encourage players to talk about any signs they have of overexertion. Experiences from the UEFA ECIS indicate that good internal communication in the team (and especially among the technical staff), with an open and tolerant attitude toward detection of early signs of physical or psychological complaint, seems to be the most effective way of avoiding overload problems.

**Objective monitoring** of the players can be helpful in providing extra information about possible overloading. So far, there is no consensus of how to monitor overload in footballers. The problem is that loading prescription is often based on external factors (duration, frequency, and intensity of training) and the internal load for each player can vary considerably for the same exercise.

## 1.4.8 Methods Designed to Address Team Factors

The concept of team factors being correlated to injuries is new and not yet scientifically fully evaluated. According to the experience and opinions from the medical teams in the UEFA ECIS, **improving the internal communication** in the team seems to contribute to preventing injuries at elite level. Clubs with consistently low injury rates seem to have a very good and effective internal communication between the medical team and the coaching staff and also with the CEO and board/president of the club. At elite level, good communication often means daily meetings between staff, and discussions of the players and their injuries and performance status. Open communication with mutual respect and confidence in each other's competence seem to be important factors.

**Consistency** of personnel is another factor to consider. Recent, yet unpublished data seem to indicate that a change of head coach or fitness coaches during an ongoing season seems to be correlated with an increase of injury risk, with the change of fitness coach being a more significant influencing factor. However, having a new coach for a new season does not seem to negatively affect the injury risk.

Whether a change of medical staff during or before a season has any effect on the injury risk is not yet evaluated, but basic preventive action should involve trying to avoid changes of nonplaying staff during the season.

**Involvement of the club doctor or the medical team in signing of new players** is another important club factor. It is well known from studies that players with previous injuries have a higher risk of incurring new injuries. Hence, a key preventive measure for a club is to involve the club doctor and the medical team in the signing process of players.

**Increasing the economic resources for the medical team** might be a good investment since the loss in economy and performance is substantial for injured players at the elite level. The average cost for a first team UCL player being injured for 1 month is reported to be around 600,000 Euros.[4]

## 1.4.9 Methods Designed to Address Rules and Equipment Factors

These factors are ruled by the IFAB, but suggestions are forwarded by FIFA when it is considered that a rule change might be necessary. Both FIFA and UEFA have regulations aimed to protect the health of players, which are based on both medical research and practical experience. Attention has been directed toward fair play, which is also part of UEFA's approach to ethics. As an example, Andersen et al[42] reported how violations of the laws of the game contribute to injury. By video analyses, they also showed that the most frequent injury mechanism behind head injuries was elbow-to-head contact where the elbow was used actively at or above shoulder level. They suggested stricter rule enforcement concerning elbow use in order to reduce the risk of head injury, a reinforcement that was later adapted by FIFA and UEFA.[43]

The key to prevent injuries correlated with rules and equipment is to provide FIFA and UEFA with knowledge gained from research, as well as experiences from medical teams working in the field.

> **STEP 4: TEST-IDEAL CONDITIONS**
>
> This step is carried out in research studies, preferably in controlled trials where the preventive measures are compared with controls not using such measures. These studies evaluate the efficacy of the preventive measures under ideal circumstances. They provide research outcomes rather than true practical guidelines, but nevertheless such an evaluation is important to establish before the measures can be recommended to the football family and implemented via practical work in the field.[10]

## STEP 5: IMPLEMENTATION

The fact that preventive measures are proven to be effective in scientific studies does not mean that they work in real life on the football field.[9] The measures have to be successfully implemented within a team environment. If the team are unable or not willing to use the measures that the medical team suggests, then the preventive efforts will fail.[7] To progress from scientific results to practical application, practical tools are needed to bridge the gap between research and practice.[9] At elite level, team doctors and members of the medical teams usually closely follow developments in football medicine and are well informed about preventive measures. However, team doctors and medical teams are not in control of, or do not always have influence on, the majority of factors behind injuries. It is therefore a challenging, but very important, task to convince players and other team officials to participate and cooperate in preventive actions.

The key is internal communication and motivation. Doctors have to convince the team staff of the benefits of injury prevention measures and keeping the players on the pitch, and this has to be done in a simple and engaging format. To get the attention from other team staff and officials, medical information has to be transformed into tactical or economical information. Informing about the relationship between injuries and performance, or about the economic cost of injuries, usually gets attention.

A doctor might come across many obstacles when attempting to implement preventive measures. One could be a concern from coaches about the lack of football specificity, or validity of the preventive measures. For the modern coach, football specificity is essential and training sessions must mimic matches in intensity and movement. Consequently, preventive measures involving static movements or movements not mimicking match play might be less attractive for coaches. A further obstacle might be the lack of time. Many elite-level clubs have a very congested calendar[25] with many matches to play and prepare for, as well as many days of travel. Such a match schedule has a negative effect on the availability of training sessions and for obvious reasons, coaches might be reluctant to include time-consuming preventive measures in their training schedule. Another obstacle might be negative opinions from players. Players might consider preventive training boring and even complain about side effects like soreness of muscles.

## STEP 6: COMPLIANCE

The aim of compliance is to achieve high-quality participation and cooperation between clubs/national associations, coaches, medical teams, and players.

The effectiveness of an injury prevention program depends on the acceptance and uptake of the intervention among participants, in other words, their compliance.[36,44] Knowledge about the relationship between compliance and injury prevention effectiveness is limited. Players with high compliance appear to benefit in terms of fewer injuries.[36] Positive coach attitudes are associated with high compliance and lower injury risk.[36] According to studies by Soligard et al,[36] coaches who previously in their career have used injury preventive training have lower injury rates in their teams compared with teams of coaches who had not used such training. The findings underline the importance of the coaching staff in influencing the injury situation within a team.

## STEP 7: SURVEILLANCE (DID IT WORK IN REAL LIFE?)

This is the final step, and is a test of whether the preventive measures are effective when applied in the real football world. The ideal of course would be if scientifically proven preventive measures (according to step 4) could be tested in controlled trials on the field (**Fig. 1.7**). However, carrying out controlled trials with elite-level players is very difficult. In real life, a more practical way for a team to evaluate the effectiveness of new preventive measures is to compare the injury statistics for the club before and after the introduction of the preventive measures. A prerequisite for doing this is to use a reliable and consistent method of injury data collection (such as the data collection method used in the UEFA ECIS, the method and forms being available from UEFA).

## 1.5 Are We Successful in Keeping the Players on the Pitch?

The answer is yes at amateur and youth level, but no with regard to elite level. Several studies on youth and amateur level have shown preventive programs

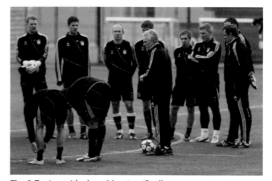

**Fig. 1.7**   In an ideal world, scientifically proven preventive measures would be tested in controlled trials on the field.

to be effective at the step 4 level[5,35,45] as well as at the step 7 level.[36] The main focus of these programs have been on player factors, and in providing the players with some sort of training program.

There are no studies on preventive measures on male senior elite level in football. A reason for this could be the difficulty in carrying out randomized studies at elite level. An indirect way of studying the effect of preventive efforts is to study time trends of injuries. In the UEFA ECIS, the highest ranked teams in Europe have been followed prospectively for many years. An 11-year follow-up showed a decreasing injury rate of ligament injuries (especially ankle injuries and medial collateral ligament injuries but not ACL injuries) which could be an effect of preventive measures.[2,46,47] However, the total injury rates showed no tendency to diminish and the most common single injury type, the hamstring muscle injury, was even increasing in spite of all efforts made to prevent injuries (**Fig. 1.8**).[2]

These findings indicate that the traditional injury prevention methods used (mainly focusing on player factors) might not be enough at the elite level. There could be several reasons for this. One reason could be that at elite level, players are indeed elite athletes and they already have strong stamina (being strong, quick, coordinated, and well trained). Furthermore, at elite level, player factors might not be the most important risk factors. Load factors and club factors might be more important, indicating that other team staff and officials could have more influence than the medical team on the injury pattern in a team.[4]

## 1.6 Conclusions

The key aspects of injury prevention can be summarized as below:
- Existing preventive methods are not effective enough at the elite level.
- Injury rates are still unacceptably high.
- Those working in football medicine need to be more open to the wide range of factors that can potentially influence injury.

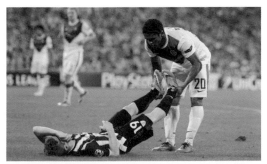

**Fig. 1.8** Traditional injury prevention methods might not be enough at the elite level.

- Good internal communication between the medical team and other members of the team staff is essential.
- Coaches should be encouraged wherever possible to understand the potential value of medical developments to performance. It is the medical teams' job to identify relevant data and to present it to the coach in a clear, concise, and meaningful way
- Medical teams need to be more football specific, to be football doctors, not just doctors.

For the team doctor, it is not possible to control all the external factors that may influence injury, but raising awareness of the range of factors within the team, and identifying practical implications, particularly in relation to performance, could have a significant impact on the overall reduction of injury rates. For players and the team, the obvious outcome is a lower injury rate and potentially improved results on the field.

## References

[1] Drawer S, Fuller CW. Evaluating the level of injury in English professional football using a risk based assessment process. Br J Sports Med. 2002; 36(6):446–451

[2] Ekstrand J, Hägglund M, Kristenson K, Magnusson H, Waldén M. Fewer ligament injuries but no preventive effect on muscle injuries and severe injuries: an 11-year follow-up of the UEFA Champions League injury study. Br J Sports Med. 2013; 47(12):732–737

[3] Hägglund M, Waldén M, Magnusson H, Kristenson K, Bengtsson H, Ekstrand J. Injuries affect team performance negatively in professional football: an 11-year follow-up of the UEFA Champions League injury study. Br J Sports Med. 2013; 47(12):738–742

[4] Ekstrand J. Keeping your top players on the pitch: The key to football medicine at a professional level. Br J Sports Med. 2013; 47 (12):723–724

[5] Ekstrand J, Gillquist J, Liljedahl SO. Prevention of soccer injuries. Supervision by doctor and physiotherapist. Am J Sports Med. 1983; 11 (3):116–120

[6] van Mechelen W, Hlobil H, Kemper HC. Incidence, severity, aetiology and prevention of sports injuries. A review of concepts. Sports Med. 1992; 14(2):82–99

[7] Finch C. A new framework for research leading to sports injury prevention. J Sci Med Sport. 2006; 9(1–2):3–9, discussion 10

[8] Van Tiggelen D, Wickes S, Stevens V, Roosen P, Witvrouw E. Effective prevention of sports

1

injuries: a model integrating efficacy, efficiency, compliance and risk-taking behaviour. Br J Sports Med. 2008; 42(8):648–652

[9] Verhagen E, Voogt N, Bruinsma A, Finch CF. A knowledge transfer scheme to bridge the gap between science and practice: an integration of existing research frameworks into a tool for practice. Br J Sports Med. 2014; 48(8):698–701

[10] Verrelst R. The role of proximal risk factors in the development of exertional medial tibial pain: A prospective study. PhD thesis. University of Ghent, the Netherlands, University of Ghent; 2014

[11] Fuller CW, Ekstrand J, Junge A, et al. Consensus statement on injury definitions and data collection procedures in studies of football (soccer) injuries. Br J Sports Med. 2006; 40 (3):193–201

[12] Hägglund M, Waldén M, Bahr R, Ekstrand J. Methods for epidemiological study of injuries to professional football players: developing the UEFA model. Br J Sports Med. 2005; 39 (6):340–346

[13] Arnason A, Sigurdsson SB, Gudmundsson A, Holme I, Engebretsen L, Bahr R. Risk factors for injuries in football. Am J Sports Med. 2004; 32 (1) Suppl:5S–16S

[14] Kristenson K, Waldén M, Ekstrand J, Hägglund M. Lower injury rates for newcomers to professional soccer: a prospective cohort study over 9 consecutive seasons. Am J Sports Med. 2013; 41(6):1419–1425

[15] Ekstrand J, Hägglund M, Waldén M. Epidemiology of muscle injuries in professional football (soccer). Am J Sports Med. 2011; 39 (6):1226–1232

[16] Hägglund M, Waldén M, Ekstrand J. Risk factors for lower extremity muscle injury in professional soccer: the UEFA Injury Study. Am J Sports Med. 2013; 41(2):327–335

[17] Ekstrand J, Torstveit MK. Stress fractures in elite male football players. Scand J Med Sci Sports. 2012; 22(3):341–346

[18] Hägglund M, Waldén M, Ekstrand J. Previous injury as a risk factor for injury in elite football: a prospective study over two consecutive seasons. Br J Sports Med. 2006; 40 (9):767–772

[19] Gajhede-Knudsen M, Ekstrand J, Magnusson H, Maffulli N. Recurrence of Achilles tendon injuries in elite male football players is more common after early return to play: an 11-year follow-up of the UEFA Champions League injury study. Br J Sports Med. 2013; 47 (12):763–768

[20] Hägglund M, Zwerver J, Ekstrand J. Epidemiology of patellar tendinopathy in elite male soccer players. Am J Sports Med. 2011; 39 (9):1906–1911

[21] Ekstrand J, van Dijk CN. Fifth metatarsal fractures among male professional footballers: a potential career-ending disease. Br J Sports Med. 2013; 47(12):754–758

[22] Ekstrand J, Karlsson J, Hodson A. Football medicine. London: Martin Dunitz (Taylor & Francis Group); 2003(Series Editor)

[23] Ascensão A, Rebelo A, Oliveira E, Marques F, Pereira L, Magalhães J. Biochemical impact of a soccer match - analysis of oxidative stress and muscle damage markers throughout recovery. Clin Biochem. 2008; 41(10–11):841–851

[24] Fatouros IG, Chatzinikolaou A, Douroudos II, et al. Time-course of changes in oxidative stress and antioxidant status responses following a soccer game. J Strength Cond Res. 2010; 24(12):3278–3286

[25] Ekstrand J, Waldén M, Hägglund M. A congested football calendar and the wellbeing of players: correlation between match exposure of European footballers before the World Cup 2002 and their injuries and performances during that World Cup. Br J Sports Med. 2004; 38 (4):493–497

[26] Richmond LK, Dawson B, Stewart G, Cormack S, Hillman DR, Eastwood PR. The effect of interstate travel on the sleep patterns and performance of elite Australian Rules footballers. J Sci Med Sport. 2007; 10(4):252–258

[27] Dellal A, Lago-Penas C, Rey E, et al. The effects of a congested fixture period on physical performance, technical activity and injury rate during matches in a professional soccer team. Br J Sports Med. 2015; 49(6):390–394

[28] Dupont G, Nedelec M, McCall A, McCormack D, Berthoin S, Wisløff U. Effect of 2 soccer matches in a week on physical performance and injury rate. Am J Sports Med. 2010; 38 (9):1752–1758

[29] Bengtsson H, Ekstrand J, Waldén M, Hägglund M. Match injury rates in professional soccer vary with match result, match venue, and type of competition. Am J Sports Med. 2013; 41 (7):1505–1510

[30] Ekstrand J, Gillquist J, Möller M, Oberg B, Liljedahl SO. Incidence of soccer injuries and their relation to training and team success. Am J Sports Med. 1983; 11(2):63–67

[31] Ekstrand J, Hägglund M, Waldén M. Injury incidence and injury patterns in professional football: the UEFA injury study. Br J Sports Med. 2011; 45(7):553–558

[32] Ekstrand J, Nigg BM. Surface-related injuries in soccer. Sports Med. 1989; 8(1):56–62

[33] Orchard JW, Waldén M, Hägglund M, et al. Comparison of injury incidences between football teams playing in different climatic regions. Open Access J Sports Med. 2013; 4:251–260

[34] Waldén M, Hägglund M, Orchard J, Kristenson K, Ekstrand J. Regional differences in injury incidence in European professional football. Scand J Med Sci Sports. 2013; 23(4):424–430

[35] Junge A, Rösch D, Peterson L, Graf-Baumann T, Dvorak J. Prevention of soccer injuries: a prospective intervention study in youth amateur players. Am J Sports Med. 2002; 30(5):652–659

[36] Soligard T, Nilstad A, Steffen K, et al. Compliance with a comprehensive warm-up programme to prevent injuries in youth football. Br J Sports Med. 2010; 44(11):787–793

[37] Tropp H, Askling C, Gillquist J. Prevention of ankle sprains. Am J Sports Med. 1985; 13 (4):259–262

[38] Petersen J, Thorborg K, Nielsen MB, Budtz-Jørgensen E, Hölmich P. Preventive effect of eccentric training on acute hamstring injuries in men's soccer: a cluster-randomized controlled trial. Am J Sports Med. 2011; 39 (11):2296–2303

[39] Caraffa A, Cerulli G, Projetti M, Aisa G, Rizzo A. Prevention of anterior cruciate ligament injuries in soccer. A prospective controlled study of proprioceptive training. Knee Surg Sports Traumatol Arthrosc. 1996; 4(1):19–21

[40] Eriksson LI, Jorfeldt L, Ekstrand J. Overuse and distorsion soccer injuries related to the player's estimated maximal aerobic work capacity. Int J Sports Med. 1986; 7(4):214–216

[41] Ivarsson A, Johnson U, Podlog L. Psychological predictors of injury occurrence: a prospective investigation of professional Swedish soccer players. J Sport Rehabil. 2013; 22(1):19–26

[42] Andersen TE, Engebretsen L, Bahr R. Rule violations as a cause of injuries in male Norwegian professional football: are the referees doing their job? Am J Sports Med. 2004; 32(1) Suppl:62S–68S

[43] Andersen TE, Arnason A, Engebretsen L, Bahr R. Mechanisms of head injuries in elite football. Br J Sports Med. 2004; 38(6):690–696

[44] Hägglund M, Atroshi I, Wagner P, Waldén M. Superior compliance with a neuromuscular training programme is associated with fewer ACL injuries and fewer acute knee injuries in female adolescent football players: secondary analysis of an RCT. Br J Sports Med. 2013; 47 (15):974–979

[45] Waldén M, Atroshi I, Magnusson H, Wagner P, Hägglund M. Prevention of acute knee injuries in adolescent female football players: cluster randomised controlled trial. BMJ. 2012; 344: e3042

[46] Lundblad M, Waldén M, Magnusson H, Karlsson J, Ekstrand J. The UEFA injury study: 11-year data concerning 346 MCL injuries and time to return to play. Br J Sports Med. 2013; 47(12):759–762

[47] Waldén M, Hägglund M, Ekstrand J. Time-trends and circumstances surrounding ankle injuries in men's professional football: an 11-year follow-up of the UEFA Champions League injury study. Br J Sports Med. 2013; 47 (12):748–753

# Chapter 2

## Rehabilitation in Football Medicine

*Jason Palmer*

**2**

## 2.1 Introduction

The goal of this chapter is to introduce concepts and a framework that can be applied to the rehabilitation of football injuries. It is based on a multidisciplinary approach of graduated functional movement to progress the player. Importantly this framework is one that can be adapted to any environment. It does not require a great deal of equipment, aims to keep things very simple, and therefore can be implemented by any football medicine department staff member.

> **NOTE:**
> "You don't need to be, or have been a good footballer, to do good football rehab."

Unfortunately, there is no single magic treatment that can be successfully applied to every injury. All injuries are different and each football medicine department will differ dramatically in how it delivers its service. This chapter provides a framework on which doctors can build and adapt their rehab approach to be specific to their own team environment. First, some concepts about organizational approaches and philosophies of rehabilitation are considered. Then, the specific variables around which rehab should develop are introduced. Appendix 0 offers a set of drills that any football doctor can start using immediately in their everyday work, and develop further as required.

## 2.2 The Football Medicine Department and Rehabilitation

Ultimately, the goal of every staff member of a football club, regardless of which department they work in, is to help their team win trophies. Championships are won by winning games and therefore the best thing a football medicine department can do to assist players, the club, its coach/manager, and the team to win games is to have the maximum number of players fit and available for selection. Greater player availability for selection gives coaches/managers the greatest potential to select their best team, and research has shown that teams with the best player availability over a season tend to win trophies (European Union of Football Associations Elite Club Injury Study [UEFA ECIS]).

Effective rehabilitation of injury (i.e., returning players to the training environment) is one of the most important contributions a football medicine department can make to a club. Most would agree that the rehabilitation process in football medicine includes those assessments, treatments, and interventions that aim to facilitate the process of optimal recovery from injury, illness, or disease and therefore permit a player to return to play. However, the whole process of delivering effective rehabilitation is more than just what happens from the time of injury. The processes, procedures, and protocols in place within a department are also key aspects of effective rehabilitation, as they will govern how a player and his/her injury is approached and managed, and also the format of the rehabilitation interventions.

## 2.3 Where Do You Start When You Want to Deliver Effective Football Rehabilitation?

A correct diagnosis is essential to the rehabilitation process. Without it, treatments and interventions do not have a focus. Effective rehabilitation also requires good preparation and planning. Therefore, an important place to start is to understand your resources, the expectations placed on you, and what procedures, processes, and protocols you have available to use, or need to develop, before you are confronted with an injury.

Below are just some of the things you might want to know or should establish before you start your rehabilitation service.

- What staff do you have available to you and what are their skills?
- What equipment and facilities do you have available to you and what do you need?
- What are the main types of injuries you will need to rehabilitate?
- What audit do you have of the rehabilitation currently being performed?
- What do your coach, club, and players expect from the rehabilitation process?
- How are you going to communicate information about the rehabilitation process?
- Who is going to communicate, and to whom?
- How will your team approach the rehab process?
- How will you judge the effectiveness of the process?

The answers to these questions will help form an important part of the rehabilitation framework and philosophy. Having a clear understanding is essential to ensure effective rehabilitation.

## 2.4 Your Resources

### 2.4.1 Human Resources: A Team's Greatest Resource

Few would challenge the value of a multidisciplinary team (MDT) approach to the effective assessment and rehabilitation of a sports injury.

Therefore, it is important to understand what staff you have and what their skills are. The makeup of the team will vary from club to club and the way the team works will mean different members of the team will have differing contributions to this process at different times. The important thing is that team members have a clear understanding of their role and the departmental procedures.

> **NOTE:**
>
> "Ask your staff what they feel they can offer to the rehab process."

Another aspect that a team needs to understand is that different injuries will be managed in different ways by different people, and staff need to feel comfortable when they are heavily involved and when they are not. Different team members will also have different contributions to the process in terms of the decision-making process, but it should be reinforced that everyone's opinion is important. **Fig. 2.1a, b** show how for two different injuries individual staff members' contributions can vary. The key in this situation is to make sure all staff understand that on occasion contributions will vary and that what is important is the outcome for the team, not *who does what* for a player. Staff need to also make sure their personal relationship with a player does not influence the medical team's plan. They need to recognize that they will all be involved in the discussion about the rehab plan and therefore all have a degree of ownership for the whole program, even if they are not working much with the player.

> **NOTE:**
>
> "It's about the results of the team, not the results of individuals in the team."

### 2.4.2 Support Human Resources

An important part of any medical department's human resources are the external medical specialists and consultants that provide support to your team. It is incredibly important to build a strong relationship with people such as orthopaedic surgeons, radiologists, and other medical specialists so that you can access them quickly, can trust their opinions, and know that they will "*work with you*" on each case to understand the different possible influences on decisions to be made. Key to this relationship is the fact that consultants see they are a *support service* to your department and that they are there to work "**for**" you.

In the end it will be **you who is responsible for the players' rehab**, so **YOU** need to be comfortable with the plan of action, and you should always be confident to ask questions without fear of offending. Sometimes, for example, the clinical presentation will not match the information that is identified radiologically. The most effective process to manage this situation is for medical staff to discuss with those reporting on investigations what the injury history and clinical findings are before the specialist writes a report. This way the radiologist, for example, has as much information as possible on which to comment on the investigation. Investigations sometimes identify abnormalities that are not relevant to the current injury, and this information can lead the rehabilitation in the wrong direction. To effectively manage this situation, your relationship with your radiologist

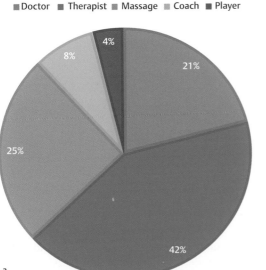

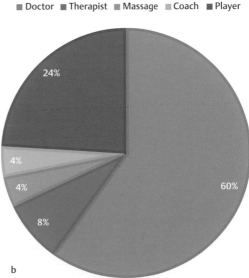

**Fig. 2.1** **(a)** Example staff contributions to a rehabilitation program for two possible different injuries. **(b)** Example staff contributions to a rehabilitation program for two possible different injuries.

2

needs to be such that you can explain what the clinical presentation is and focus on things related to that clinical information, making note of, but not placing a focus on, the other less relevant radiological findings.

| NOTE:

"With time YOU will be the football medicine expert, so ask questions of your fellow medical professionals to help clarify the diagnosis clearly."

There are many specialities that you may need to access over a season to manage the injuries and illnesses of a football team. It is unlikely you will be able to build a close relationship with members of all these specialities; therefore, you may choose to have a lead consultant who can act as your direct pathway to the other medical specialists. This consultant should be someone who you are in contact with more often than others and also preferably someone well connected in the local medical infrastructure. By making this professional an important and valued member of your team, you will find the process of accessing other specialists is made both simpler and more efficient.

## 2.5 Equipment and Facilities

### 2.5.1 What Resources Do You Have, and What Do You Need?

When you have a good understanding of the people in your team and their skills, it is important to then evaluate what equipment, resources, and facilities you have access to. These are the things you and your fellow staff members will use to deliver the rehabilitation treatments and interventions.

Below are some example questions you might consider:

- Where will you perform the assessments (e.g., which room, is it private and quiet?)?

- Do you have a stock of basic medication, splints, braces, etc., that you would regularly use?
- If you require investigations, where is the nearest facility? How easily can you get an appointment and how much will it cost?
- What treatment equipment do you have? What equipment do you need?
- Can you access a grass pitch and some basic equipment for the functional rehab at any time?
- Do you have access to a pool?
- Do you have access to strengthening equipment, or a gym?
- What is the medical budget and the department's financial constraints?
- What other resources will you need to manage the majority of injuries you will confront?

It is important that you are constantly looking to see how you can improve the quality of rehabilitation your department delivers. At first, you may not be able to add to your resources due to budgetary restraints, but being aware of what you feel would help you deliver better results, and what your priorities would be if you can develop the department further, will make it easier for you to act when the opportunity presents itself to grow.

## 2.6 Developing Your Treatment Options Framework

Once you know what skills and equipment you have available, it can be useful to develop a treatment options framework to reference at the start of any rehabilitation plan. Such a framework can be an invaluable tool at the start of every rehabilitation plan and will save time and thought. **Fig. 2.2** shows an example of a basic framework for the injury rehab planning process. Every team's framework will differ because it will reflect what equipment and staff

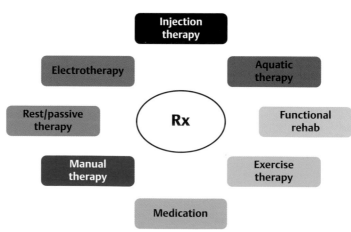

**Fig. 2.2** Example of Stage 1 of a treatment option framework.

skills they have available. It is also important to remember that not **all** treatment options will be used every time. Sometimes you need to be selective about using the ones that are most appropriate for the situation. Factors that can effect these selections can be the player's current injury, their previous experiences with rehab, the staff working with the player, the time you have available, and what access you have to equipment and facilities.

Once you have your general treatment options identified (i.e., Stage 1), you can develop the framework further. This process involves taking one of your Stage 1 variables and defining what specific treatments or forms it can take. In **Fig. 2.3**, you can see how the Exercise Therapy variable has been broken down further into types of exercise therapy (e.g., isokinetic exercise, isometric exercise, isotonic exercise). The Electrotherapy variable has also been broken down into potential types of devices available for use. By investing time early in thinking about your options before you need to deal with an injury, you will save yourself time when planning.

For some Stage 1 variables, there may not be a Stage 2 level, e.g., Medication (see **Fig. 2.4**). Most variables, however, will have more specific levels you can identify and therefore the process can be continued until

you have been specific enough to see what treatment options you have.

This process of documenting the options you have available will start in a very basic form and can be developed over time. Having such a framework, and importantly having staff contribute to its development, can also mean a consistent planning process across the department and club, such that no matter who does the planning, the program will be similar.

## 2.7 Planning

> **NOTE:**
>
> "The key to success in football rehabilitation is good planning."

### 2.7.1 Daily Planning

Having a general treatment plan for your department to use on a daily basis improves organization and helps communicate responsibility and focus, therefore using time more efficiently. By having such a Daily Treatment Plan available for *all* to see, injured players feel like time has been invested in their rehab, structure is given to both the players' and staff

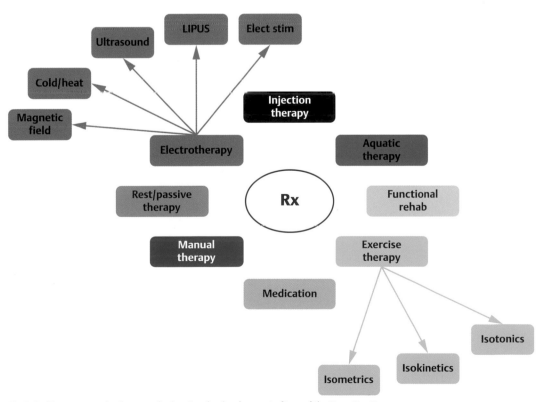

**Fig. 2.3**  Treatment option framework, showing the development of two of the Stage 2 options.

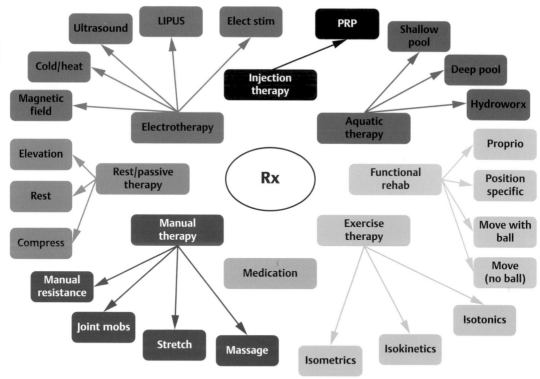

**Fig. 2.4**  Stage 2 treatment option framework.

members' days, and it also provides a good reference for further planning.

One option is to have a brief meeting at the end of each day to develop a Daily Treatment Plan for the following day. This can be useful to engage all those in the rehab process, and to allow staff to share their thoughts and reflections. This Daily Treatment Plan documents general information about injured players' rehab content and also squad training information, so, for example, staff can be kept free for fit players immediately before and after training.

A modified traffic light system to reflect on players' relative fitness is one method to consider for the whole squad. Players are considered as being **red, yellow, or green**. Fit players who are training and have no injury or "niggle" of any sort are identified as being "green." These players do not require much attention during the day other than perhaps aspects of their normal routine such as an ankle strapping before training. Players that are injured are classified as "red." They have an individually structured day (see Players 1, 2, and 3 in **Fig. 2.5**). Finally, those players who are training but report having a "niggle" which requires some attention, or players recently back from injury who need some additional monitoring or treatment, are classified as "yellow." The "yellow" players (see players 4, 5, and 6 in **Fig. 2.5**)

are listed on the Daily Treatment Plan just to make staff aware that they require some attention, even if that attention is asking how they felt in training.

The goal should be to keep players training and therefore trying to prevent the "*greens*" turning into "*yellows*" and perhaps more importantly, trying to prevent the "*yellows*" turning into "*reds*."

The Daily Treatment Plan in **Fig. 2.5** shows how staff members have their own color, so that players can easily see who they should be with, where they should be, and what time they should be there. As mentioned earlier, the majority of staff are kept free immediately before and after training so that fit players can access the medical staff for any maintenance treatment, reviews, or simply some assistance stretching, or for a massage. In some clubs, a member of staff with emergency training attends each training session in case of an accident or injury. On this day, you can see it is the doctor who is covering training.

Each morning before any players arrive, the medical team working that day can meet for 5 to 10 minutes to review what issues the players reported the day before, discuss any new "yellows," etc., and review the Daily Treatment Plan for that day. This way everyone knows what they and their colleagues are doing for that day. Staff need to work hard to stick

| Wednesday 3rd December | | | | | | | | |
|---|---|---|---|---|---|---|---|---|
| Name | Player1 | Player2 | Player3 | | | | | |
| Start time | | | | | | | | |
| 09:30 | Review | | | | | | | |
| 09:45 | Treatment | | | | | | | |
| 10:00 | Bike | | | | | | | |
| 10:15 | Stretch | | | | | | | |
| 10:30 | Outside Session | Review | | | | Yellows | | Training |
| 10:45 | | Treatment | | | | Player 4 | | Doctor |
| 11:00 | | " | | | | Player 5 | | " |
| 11:15 | | Pool | | | | Player 6 | | " |
| 11:30 | Pool Recovery | " | | | | | | " |
| 11:45 | Contrast Bath | Ice bath | | | | | | |
| 12:00 | Magnetic Field | Ultrasound | | | | | | |
| 12:15 | Ice | Ice | | | | | | |
| 12:30 | Lunch | Lunch | Depart | | | | | |
| 12:45 | " | " | | | | | | |
| 13:00 | Electrical Stim | Magnetic Field | MRI Scan | | | | | |
| 13:30 | Treatment | " | " | | | | | |
| 13:45 | " | Treatment | " | | | | | |
| 14:00 | Bike/Stretch | " | " | | | | | |
| 14:15 | Isokinetic Session | Bike | Pod | | | Colour Code System | | |
| 14:30 | " | Proprioception | " | | | Doctor | | |
| 14:45 | Treatment | " | Ice bath | | | Physio 1 | | |
| 15:00 | " | Pool | Treatment | | | Physio 2 | | |
| 15:15 | Ice | " | " | | | Sport Therapist | | |
| 15:30 | Finish | Ice bath | UPUS (US) | | | Massage Therapist | | |
| 15:45 | | Compression | Ice | | | Player is self supervised | | |
| 16:00 | | Finish | Magnetic Field | | | | | |
| 16:15 | | | " | | | | | |
| 16:30 | | | Massage | | | | | |
| 16:45 | | | Ice | | | | | |
| 17:00 | | | | | | | | |

**Fig. 2.5**  Example of a daily treatment plan.

with the plan, and must be on time and be ready for the players so that they see a professional approach from the staff.

It is important to remember to never overlook the needs of the fit players, as they are the ones going out on the pitch in the next game. By checking up on the "yellow players" and treating their "niggles," often these niggles can be resolved or reduced and the player never becomes a "red" and so could be seen as a type of injury prevention.

**NOTE:**

"Training is the best prevention for injuries."

Injury prevention has long been the aspiration of many medical departments, as it is surely better to prevent the injury rather than cure it. There are many ways to approach prevention programs, and discussion in depth on this topic is beyond the scope of this chapter. What is worth mentioning, however, is that the philosophy being proposed here is that the goal of rehabilitation in football is to get a player back to training as fast and as safely as possible. Training is the most specific activity available that replicates match play. Since we know that the best injury prevention programs are specific to the sporting activity, getting a player back to training as soon as possible

means they are performing specific functional activity in the specific environment sooner. It could be said therefore that the best prevention program is training itself. Training is also the final stage of a rehabilitation program, as it almost impossible to replicate the reactive movements and awareness that are required in a training session. Therefore, as a prevention program, a logical but progressive return to training following injury is certainly useful. Worth also noting is that the coaching staff need to recognize that the player coming back into training following injury can have some associated risks, so it would be wise to not challenge them maximally in their first session.

## 2.8 Prognosis

**NOTE:**

"How long will I be out Doc?"

Every doctor has been asked at some stage, normally within minutes of an injury, and before they have even assessed a player, "How long will I be out Doc?" This question can put pressure on staff to provide a timescale and then stick to it.

The reality is that all players are different, their rate of recovery from injury is different, and their injuries are different, so it can be difficult to accurately predict rehabilitation times. When you say an injury will take 4 weeks to recover and it ends up being 5 weeks, and you get negative feedback and increased pressure as a result; next time you think it is a 4-week injury, you may say 5 weeks to protect yourself and the department from criticism. Therefore, a logical approach to rehab prognosis is necessary, along with a strong communication path with your coach and the players. Trust is essential for this to succeed.

When, for example, an injury occurs and it is suspected on the basis of the diagnosis that the player will "on average" be back to training in around 3 weeks, then a player could be told the shortest possible time they *may* recover in, which for this example might be 2 weeks. The reason this could be proposed is that if 3 weeks is proposed, then the earliest it will be will be 3 weeks, as everyone including the player will work to this time frame. If it is proposed to get the player back at the earliest possible time, then as long as the progression is logical but progressive, time landmarks do not become the focus, and it gives the player and the injury a chance to recover faster if possible. Sometimes players do return earlier than expected because everyone is thinking and working to get them back as soon as they are ready.

Essential to this approach is that the coach/manager, the player, the staff, and the club understand the rationale behind approaching the prognosis in this way. With good, consistent results however and an honest approach, trust will be generated. When all see that the goal is to get players back as soon as is safely possible, few will challenge you.

When using this approach, it is important to mention a few things that are essential to this philosophy. At the time of providing a prognosis, tell the player that "**at no time during the rehab are they expected to tolerate or push through any pain or discomfort.**" Tell them that you will "**get them moving as soon as they are ready**" and that you are aiming to get them back to training as soon as possible. Also, say that "**if they need more time, that's ok.**" Reassure them that you will take the time needed to get them right, but you are not going to delay the process unnecessarily. The progression will be based on what they can do, not the calendar or the prognosis for that matter.

> **NOTE:**
> "Rehab should be pain free, and based on the clinical presentation."

With this approach, it is hard for a player to not agree with the plan. In the end, you are offering him/her a pain-free path back to training as soon as possible, which is what most players want.

Above we noted that the manager/coach needs to understand and agree with this approach. It is therefore preferable if you are not criticized if the player returns at 3 weeks when you initially said 2 weeks. This being said, you also need to not be wrong all the time. However, with practice and some experience, your results will be consistent and you can be more confident of your prognosis.

Medical professionals working in football aim to get players back as soon as possible without unnecessary risk of reinjury. Reinjury though does happen and it could be said that if you have never had a reinjury or a setback, then you may be overly conservative in your rehab. Similarly, it could be said if you are regularly getting reinjuries, you are a little too aggressive in your rehab approach. To truly understand what you are doing, you need to reflect on your results.

## 2.9 Results and Audit

> **NOTE:**
> "How do you reflect on your results?"

Having some form of audit of your results allows you to see how your department performs. Reflecting on this information will help enhance your prognosis skills and will allow you to compare your results. These comparisons can be to your own previous years' results, or you can compare your results with others treating similar injuries in a similar environment, such as through published audits like the UEFA ECIS. There are various software packages that are available to assist you to generate statistics about your rehab, or you can do the analysis yourself. If, however, you are not reflecting on what you are doing, it is hard to know what you did well and what may not have gone so well.

Having an audit system is also very useful when you come to communicate with your coach/manager, club, and its hierarchy. Having a valid system that shows how your department performs can help provide some evidence or a rational for proposals for more staff, for example, or for more equipment.

With respect to your injury audit, the best outcome you can hope for is to have consistent results where you are getting players back promptly. The cornerstone of this process is a good diagnosis. If your diagnosis is incorrect, you start on the wrong path from day 1 and are therefore wasting time, so it is worth investing time in getting it right.

## 2.10 Diagnosis

Rehabilitation is a little like a jigsaw puzzle. You need to begin with something you believe is correct, and then build on from there until the puzzle is complete. The first piece of the puzzle in rehabilitation is the diagnosis. The correct diagnosis is essential to start you thinking and acting in the right direction. A correct diagnosis can be achieved with accurate history taking, effective assessment skills, and a united approach from the medical team.

At the time of the initial complete assessment, the injured player should be taken to a private area. This shows the player that you are interested and focused on their problem. It also allows an injured player to speak more freely, and avoids other players who may be present from providing their opinion on the issue. Involve as many members of the medical team in this process as available. This again shows the player that they are important, that the medical team are united, and it ensures all staff members are part of the decision making process. This point is very important, as being part of the group decision-making process implies a degree of ownership of that decision, and should ensure the medical team have *one* opinion and the same voice that says the same thing no matter which staff member is asked.

In a MDT approach, different members with the appropriate skills and training will benefit from having a chance to take the lead in the subjective and physical examination. This process is good for staff members' confidence, contributes to their professional development, and again reinforces the team approach to the player. If a member of the staff is not leading the examination, but wants to know further information or assess something themselves, then they should feel free to do so once the "lead" has finished and looks to his/her colleagues for anything further that they might want to consider or examine. One thing to be careful about, however, is to not overdiagnose. Gather the information you require to make the diagnosis but try to keep the process simple and brief if possible. Once you have a "good feel for the problem," stop. Normally you will see the player regularly and can gather further detailed information over time.

Once the examination has been completed, and before discussing the diagnosis with the player, explain to them that the medical staff will first discuss the injury together and will then discuss the diagnosis with the player. Explain that this is the same for all injuries, so the player does not become alarmed, and be sure to be consistent with this practice where possible. At this point, either request that the player leave the room if they are sufficiently mobile or the staff can leave the room.

Once in private, staff should discuss what they feel the issue is and why. All staff should have an opportunity to contribute and offer their opinion. Everyone will not always agree, which is actually healthy for the success of the process, as long as all understand that this process is not personal, but professional and should be based on the information determined in the assessment. When the group leaves that discussion room and goes to talk with the player, all must agree to conform to the group decision. Staff members who contradict the group decision after that discussion can undermine the department and weaken the strength of the department, so try to involve staff and make sure they understand the process.

It is important in an effective MDT approach that all members understand and respect each other's area of expertise and knowledge, that all members understand that one person does not always have the answer, that the loudest is not always right, that it is ok to suggest something that is incorrect, and that sometimes the conclusions made by the team will be wrong. No medical team in football always gets it right. Having more minds reflecting on the information together, however, gives the process greater strength. Also if the group are constantly reflecting on the player's presentation and relating it back to the diagnosis during the rehab process, it will soon become evident that the current diagnosis may not be 100% accurate and can be adjusted accordingly.

## 2.11 Documenting the Injury

### 2.11.1 Injury Cards

An injury card system can be useful during the process of assessment to document information gathered regarding a player and a new injury. An example injury card is shown in **Fig. 2.6**. The information documented is based around items that may be useful at some stage in the rehabilitation process. The value of completing an injury card is that it can:

— Provide a point of reference for relevant information regarding the injury.
— Permit quick reflection at a later point when reviewing players.
— Help other staff not present during the initial assessment to see what the team thinks so far and what conclusions were made.
— Prompt the gathering of all relevant information that may have been forgotten.
— Act as a guide for team members on treatment planning.
— Document the "team's" information, highlighting the department's MDT approach.

These documents should be individual to your team and should include information that you may want

2

# Injury Card

| Player Name: | | Injury Date: | (Match)    Training    Other |
|---|---|---|---|
| PLAYER X. | | 13/09/14 | Minutes.....6.7..... |
| **Mechanism of Injury:** | | | Video Clip:   (Yes)  No |
| BLOCK TACKLE WITH ®️ LEG | | | STRONG VALGUS FORCE |

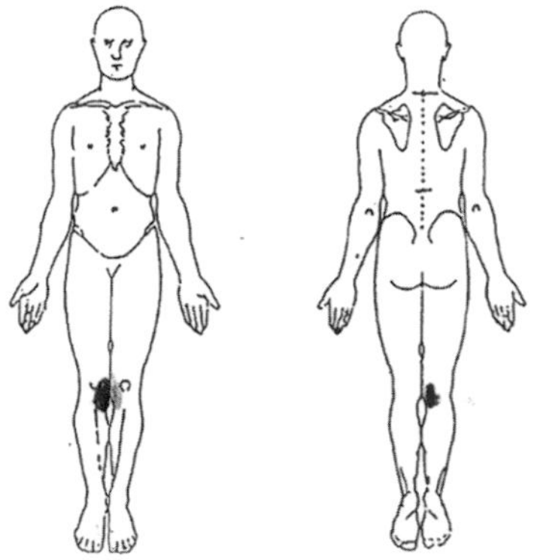

**Clinical Findings:**

- PAIN WITH PALPATION + MOVT ®️ MCL
- KNEE FLEXION = 5-60°
- MILD LAXITY ®️ MCL
- SMALL EFFUSION, ACL + PCL ✓

**Relevant Radiology Findings:**

- MRI BOOKED FOR TOMORROW
- @ 11 AM 15/09/14.

**Diagnosis:**
- ? ®️ MCL GRADE I-II

**Medication: (include dosage, and number of days)**

- DICLOFENAC 50mg TDS. FOR 4 DAYS.
- PARACETAMOL AS REQUIRED.
- _____

**Proposed Acute Treatment: (R.I.C.E. etc.)**

- . ICE, COMPRESSION .
- 'PAIN FREE WALK IN WATER
- _____

**Other Proposed Treatment (supplements, PRP, etc)**

- ? PRP AFTER MRI TOMORROW .
- _____

**Return to Training (RTT):**

- **Proposed days to RTT** ___2 WEEKS.___
- **Key criteria for RTT** PAIN FREE VALGUS TESTING, PAIN FREE KICKING
- _____

**Fig. 2.6** Example injury card document.

to know or that will guide your practice. Detail can also be added at any time as more information becomes available (e.g., investigation reports).

## 2.12  An Injury, from Day 1

The work of a rehab program begins from the time of the diagnosis, as this is when the injury becomes more clearly understood. Sometimes, it may be 1 to 2 days after the injury before the definitive diagnosis has been agreed. The work done however between the time of the injury and the actual diagnosis to manage the player can also impact the rehabilitation process.

The following points demonstrate this by means of an example that follows an injury from the moment it occurs. During the process, reference is made to items discussed so far in the chapter, examples are used to illustrate concepts, and questions are asked to prompt you to think about what processes and procedures you may wish to have in place.

### 2.12.1  An Injury Occurs in a Match

**At the Match**
— Who is running on to the field to review the player?
  • Does more than one staff member go on? For example, doctor and physical therapist together.
  • Who takes the lead, and why?
  • What equipment are the staff members taking on with them?
— Do you have a protocol for reviewing common injuries on the pitch during the match?
  • See Appendix 0: Pitch Assessment (Ankle Protocol).
  • Who decides if a player can continue or not?
— How are you communicating to the team bench and the emergency services?
  • Visual signals or audio method via communication devices.
  • How do you call on a stretcher or further assistance?
— Do you have a procedure for removal of players off the pitch, and off to hospital.
  • Is there an ambulance on site? If not, how far away is it? How is it going to get to the best location as fast as possible?
  • Are stretcher bearers trained in basic procedures of lifting the player?
  • Can an ambulance come pitchside or on the pitch? Is the pathway locked? Who has the key?
  • What emergency equipment do you have at matches? Who is responsible for checking it is

there and working? Where is it kept? Does staff know how to use it?
  • How and where are players taken as they come off (i.e., dressing room or medical room, if going to hospital. Which one will be used and is a staff or team member going with them?)
  • Do you have a player emergency and medical information record folder to send to hospital with the player?

> **NOTE:**
> Most injuries do not require hospital review and are assessed by the team medical staff in the dressing room.

**In the Dressing Room**
— Who will assess the player in the dressing room?
— What is the acute injury management plan? What is done with the player before they leave the dressing room after the game: ice, compression, elevation, crutches, joint bracing, medication, etc.?
— What advice are you going to give the player for them to do until you see them next?
  • Ice: How often and for how long and via what method?
  • Medication: What to take and when?
  • Compression: Do they leave compression on or take it off to ice?
— When will you see them next and where?
Managing small details immediately after the match can result in the player presenting the next day in better shape, with less swelling, for example, which means you are already closer to the player's return to training.

### 2.12.2  The Day after the Injury the Player Comes in to Be Reassessed

**At the Training Ground**
— Who is involved in the assessment? MDT approach?
— How is the injury information initially documented? Do you have an injury card?
— Do you have previous injury or screening information available to refer to?
— Was there video footage available of the injury you can review?
— Who leads the assessment?
— How is the need for further imaging decided? Who decides? What imaging will you do?
— How and who is involved in the final diagnosis?
— Do you provide a prognosis? How do you determine this time frame?

2

- To whom do you need to give feedback regarding the diagnosis and prognosis?

### 2.12.3 The Diagnosis of the Injury Has Been Established and the Rehabilitation Process Can Begin

#### Acute Management of the Injury

- What do you do in the acute phase of an injury?
  - Do you have a protocol to follow?
  - Medication? Manual therapy? Electrotherapy? Aquatic therapy?
  - What techniques, equipment, and dosages are you going to use?
  - Refer to your treatment framework options and resources evaluation to determine what you can use.
  - Which staff member works with the player? Is there a lead therapist?

### 2.12.4 The Acute Phase of the Injury Is Now Passed and It Is Time to Start a Functional Progression

#### Nonweight-Bearing Function

| NOTE: |

"Pain-free movement is therapeutic."

The goal of any football rehabilitation program is for the player to return to normal function, i.e., full weight-bearing (WB). WB through an injured limb can however be very painful soon after an injury and often the player cannot function comfortably bearing weight normally. *Pain-free movement of a normal pattern is therapeutic*, so the sooner the player can start to move in a pain-free, familiar pattern, the better. Therefore, before a player tries bearing weight in any way, they should be able to and be confident to move into or at least rest the injured area in the position or range of motion necessary for the activity in question.

- For example, if a player cannot passively have his knee flexed to 10 degrees without significant pain while resting on the treatment couch, it is unlikely they will be able to flex their knee to step up a stair with full WB in a normal pattern of movement.

So if you are not sure about what they can do, assess the player on the treatment couch. This will be good for both your and their confidence. Players will gain confidence from pain-free movement via confident manual handling of their injured area. Carefully but confidently review the injured area first in isolation, supporting immediately above and below the area in question.

- For example, if the player's ankle is injured and you want to see if they can dorsiflex their ankle sufficiently to walk, rest their leg on the couch so it is supported on the bed. Support their ankle, and ask them to try to slowly move it, asking them to tell you if they feel any pain. Once you have determined the area can be moved in isolation, you can combine movement of other joints in the limb to make sure that the player and you are comfortable to introduce partial weight-bearing (PWB) exercise.

For certain injuries where you want to encourage normal or functional movement patterns and also wish to remain non-weight bearing (NWB), deep water buoyancy devices can be useful. Limbs can be moved in more normal patterns in an upright position without any WB (see **Fig. 2.7**).

#### Partial Weight-Bearing Function

Introducing normal movement patterns in a PWB environment can often accelerate the recovery of an athlete. Water is an excellent medium for this task. The deeper the player is in water, the greater is the reduction in their relative WB status due to the buoyancy effect of water. So start in deeper water if possible and then reduce the depth as comfortable to increase the relative WB percentage.

- For example, being submerged to the level of the clavicle equates to just 10 to 15% WB through the feet. Submersion to the level of the angle of the sternum equates roughly to 30% WB, and being submerged to the level at the iliac crest level approximates to 50% WB.

By starting to walk in water at 20 to 30% WB, the qualities of the water support the player and can permit a more normal walking pattern compared with trying to walk full WB in pain. For many injuries, reluctance to walk normally can be due to pain and a lack of confidence. Moving in water can be a

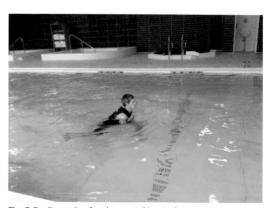

**Fig. 2.7** Example of a player working in deep water in a buoyancy vest.

great way to reduce the pain associated with WB and to build confidence in a player, which will facilitate a progression. The same concept applies to all movements. If the player can perform light multidirectional movements and run in the water with PWB, then they will be more confident when they make the transition to full WB function.

– Usually, if a player can function at 50% WB, then they make the transition to full WB with confidence.

Options for use of water range from normal pools (**Fig. 2.8**) to underwater treadmills (**Fig. 2.9**). Both have advantages and disadvantages, but finding access to water in some way and using it to progress function will help accelerate your rehabilitation.

Other methods of PWB include manual resistance on the treatment couch through the long axis of a limb and the use of antigravity treadmills through using simple crutches, where the player gradually increases the weight they are putting through a limb. Weighing scales can also be used to give the player feedback on how much weight they are putting through a limb. Water however is a superior method if it can be accessed, as it does not restrict the players' movement patterns in any direction.

Some players will not be confident swimmers or may be frightened by the prospect of getting into the water, so this needs to be taken into consideration.

## Full Weight-Bearing Function

**NOTE:**

"Getting out on the grass."

If the player has been able to do quality movement patterns in a reduced WB environment, then both you and the player will have confidence making the transition to full WB function. If you have not been able to make progress through a PWB program, then you need to introduce functional movement in its most basic form, and build up the complexity as the player tolerates each step (**Fig. 2.10**).

Below is an example of a progression from walking to jogging where a PWB progression has not been possible. This progression should be pain free:

1. Walk slowly.
2. Walk medium pace.
3. Walk and flex the hip a little more to simulate a pattern closer to jogging.
4. Walk, flex the hip a little, and rise on toes.
5. Jog on the spot with small steps using a pattern with no flight phase (one foot is always touching the ground).

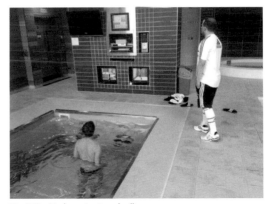

**Fig. 2.9** Underwater treadmill.

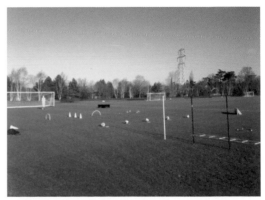

**Fig. 2.10** Build up the complexity as the player tolerates each step.

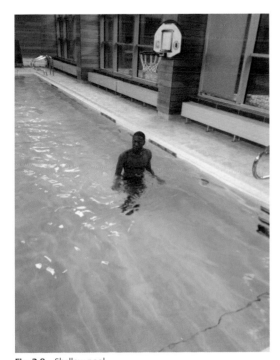

**Fig. 2.8** Shallow pool.

6. Jog with small steps moving forward slowly using a pattern with no flight phase (one foot is always touching the ground).
7. Jog with slightly longer steps so there is a flight phase (i.e., normal jogging).

Note that this progression may occur over a few sessions, over one session, or over 5 minutes. The steps are small enough such that if the player is not comfortable, then you can stay at that level and can build up a little volume before progressing. If however they can perform each stage comfortably, then progress.

Once a player can walk with full WB, then walking itself can be used as the first stage of a progression. If however, for example, a player cannot tolerate a 10-minute walk, then they are unlikely to tolerate a 10-minute session on the grass involving some jogging or light multidirectional movements, so make sure your progression has a logical rationale.

## 2.13 Planning Your Content

Once you are ready to begin on the grass, you can introduce your functional football framework progression. When thinking about the drills to use, there are several things you should think about.

### 2.13.1 How to Start
You will see that the underlying concept that is the foundation of this functional rehabilitation framework is to look at a skill or movement pattern and break it down to its most basic level. Start the player functioning at that most basic level and then build it back up again through the progression. If you start this way and progress step by step, both you and the player will be confident with the progression and you will be less likely to take too big a step. If then during your sessions you or the player is not confident to take a step, stay at the level you are working at for another day, or put in another step to help bridge the gap.

### 2.13.2 Where Do You Finish?
Something that may help you plan your overall sessions, the content, and the progression is to know where you intend to finish, i.e., what does the player need to be able to do to return to training?

If you have video footage of the injured player during a match, look at what they do as they play and then build the progression up to the point where they are performing normal football function. This is a tool that players appreciate when you can show them that you have looked at their match play and are designing their rehab specifically for them. If you do not have video footage of the player, then you can use footage of a professional player in a similar

position, one who the player aspires to play like, and compare the player to them.

## 2.14 Drill Design Variables

Below are several variables that should be taken into consideration for every drill used in a rehab session. Through understanding how to use these variables to adjust your drills, you will be able to make a drill easier or harder and more or less dynamic. This will allow you to focus on your target, so you get better quality from your sessions.

### 2.14.1 Movement

**Nature or Type of the Movement**
Although the functional movement approach aims to focus on function rather than the pathology, the nature and type of movement you are going to include in your first sessions on the grass will be influenced by the pathology you are dealing with.

It is never good to start out on the grass and walk off the pitch after 5 minutes because the player is not comfortable. Therefore, you should be confident that the player will tolerate what you plan to do, particularly in the first couple of sessions.

**NOTE:**

"Pain-free movement is therapeutic."

Players will see "*moving outside onto the grass*" as a positive step in their recovery, particularly when the injury is one that will keep them out for more than a few weeks. Therefore, a successful first session can be a significant psychological step for the player. When you plan to introduce full WB function on the grass, start with a basic level of function you are confident the player will comfortably cope with. It is also often a good idea to first introduce functional movement that does **not** specifically target the pathology. Pain-free movement is therapeutic and will build confidence, just as painful movement will undermine confidence.

For example, if you are working with a player who has an adductor injury, your first session (or at least the start of that first session) should not include anything that might stress this injury. Lateral and curved movements will challenge an adductor muscle more than straight-line work. So in the first session, you should start with linear-based movements, avoiding lateral and curved movements. The goal of your first session on the grass should be to achieve a progression in function, and for the player to complete the session you planned without any complaint of symptoms.

Worthy of note is that again as per the functional movement philosophy, as soon as you can do something you should. So if, for example, you have been doing light multidirectional movements in the water and the player has tolerated these well, then you can introduce low-intensity versions of these movements early, even in the first session.

Injury severity is also something that needs to be taken into consideration when looking at your decisions about movement content. If, for example, you have a player who has sustained a significant articular injury, and you know they will require several sessions on the grass to progress, don't push things in the first session. If however the injury was a low-grade injury like a contusion and you expect the player will progress over one to two sessions, then you will be more comfortable to progress and the player will expect to take a few steps in the first session. In this situation, the safe way to approach your sessions is to progress step by step, avoid skipping a step, and then you are unlikely to have a problem. You only need to have the player perform a "step" once and then you can take the next step. As your experience grows, you will know when you can skip a step. At first, however, be logical and progress according to a plan.

### 2.14.2 Intensity

#### Drill Intensity

The intensity of physical work performed is an important consideration for a rehabilitation progression. Initially the focus of your rehab should be the quality of the movement, not the intensity. Therefore, not surprisingly, intensity for a given type of work or drill needs to first be performed at its lowest level and then progressed as the player shows he/she can tolerate the work. A simple method to manage the intensity is to tell a player at the start of their rehab that in each session you will ask them to work at levels 1, 2, or 3. Level 1 is a light jogging pace, level 2 relates to a moderate level of intensity, and level 3 is a high to maximal level of intensity. These levels though are not discrete, and so during a session when the player has been working at level 1 and want a little more, you can say "*progress to level 1.5 but not level 2*" to explain you want a small increment of effort.

#### Session Intensity

Session intensity relates to the overall work done in a session and is influenced by the work/rest ratio of drills in a session. Again starting at the lowest level, you should focus more on movement quality than intensity, therefore using longer rest periods between drills and sets. Fatigue should not be the limiting factor early in your rehab, so if the player is challenged by the work physically, then you can give them sufficient rest to recover well between drills. For example, if a player works for 30 seconds in an early session, you may give them 60 seconds to rest between intervals. That way, fatigue won't have an influence on the quality of work. Later in the rehab progression however when you are moving toward the end of your progression, you may have the player working for 60 seconds and only give them 30 seconds to recover between intervals, which will result in a higher overall session intensity and will more closely replicate the demands of training.

### 2.14.3 Time/Volume

#### Drill Duration and Volume

The length of time needed for a drill should develop as the rehabilitation progresses. Drills at first need to be focused on quality of movement (not quantity) and therefore at first should be short (e.g., 15–20 seconds). As function improves, drill length can increase to the point where a drill may challenge a player for 2 to 3 minutes. Drills should rarely, however, require the player to work for more than 3 minutes. Football is a random interval-based game and so there is no need to work longer than this. By adjusting the rest periods between drills, you can still challenge a player physically, but still keep the session functionally specific to football.

It is also worth remembering that as a player gets close to returning to training, their function will become more dynamic and therefore of a higher intensity. In this case, you may find that the drills used in part of the session will be shorter overall, reflecting the focus on functional quality (**Fig. 2.11**).

Regarding drill repetitions and sets, it is normal to perform a drill a few times initially to allow the player to be familiar with the content, to

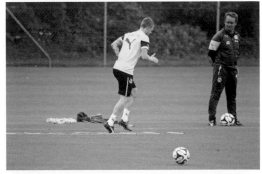

**Fig. 2.11**    As a player gets close to returning to training, their function will become more dynamic and therefore of a higher intensity.

allow you to observe them, and then also to give you the opportunity to modify the content and progress it. In one session, you may choose to include two to three sets of a drill consecutively, or you may choose to perform the drill two to three times throughout a session, having other drills in between each set. Sometimes, for example, a certain drill may contain functional movement that is the main target of the session. Subsequently, you might include this drill early in the session when the player is less fatigued, and perform two to three sets consecutively where the emphasis is on quality performance. However, your goal for a drill may just be to provide a functional volume of work for the player's condition, in which case you may include sets toward the end of the session, and therefore have more focus on *quantity* rather than quality. Just make sure you are conscious of the total volume of work done by the player in a session compared with previous sessions.

### Session Duration

Overall session time needs to be taken into consideration in conjunction with work/rest ratio times. Your first session may only last 15 minutes with rest built into the plan, but it could also last 30 to 40 minutes if you have previously spent sessions in the water, for example, that lasted a similar period of time. As your progression develops each day, you will tend to have longer sessions lasting up to 70 or 80 minutes, and the time required for resting in those sessions will tend to reduce.

If a player has been out of training for a few weeks, they need to be physically able to cope with the demand of training. So ensure that when a player is ready to be reintroduced, you are satisfied that they will cope with the way your team trains, in terms of not only intensity, but also volume.

### 2.14.4 Working Space/Distance

The size and shape of the area you work in, in combination with the intensity of the work you are doing, can significantly influence the demands placed on the player. Working in a small space at low intensity results in less challenge to a player. For example, in a small space such as a $2 \times 2$ m² space, working at level 1 intensity, the options for movement are reduced; the player cannot generate any speed or momentum and therefore there is less muscular demand on the player.

In contrast, working in a small space at a higher intensity will generate a lot of acceleration, deceleration, and agility movements, which take a lot of effort and place greater muscular demand on the body.

### 2.14.5 Reaction and Predictability

Functional rehab drill content needs to start with a more predictable and less reactive format and move toward a more reactive unpredictable format, to match the nature of training and matches. Being familiar with a drill, being aware of what the drill will demand, and being in control of functional intensity will instill confidence in a player. Having to react during a drill to unpredictable variables (e.g., doctor calls a color of a pole during a drill which the player needs to move toward) requires both movement and body confidence. Therefore, this reactive drill format should be introduced later in a progression when similar, more controlled drills have been previously performed.

### 2.14.6 Drill Complexity

Drill complexity refers to what skill content or combinations of skills you require the player to perform in any given drill. **Fig. 2.12** gives an example of a simple drill that could be introduced early in a rehab progression. Here the player moves back and forth across the ladder to volley a ball at each end, which is delivered by the therapist. **Fig. 2.13** however represents a complex drill that should be introduced late in a rehab progression as it requires more

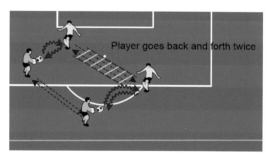

**Fig. 2.12** A simple drill format.

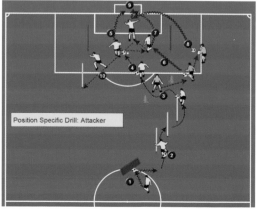

**Fig. 2.13** A complex drill format.

complex movement combinations at greater performance intensity.

Drill complexity within a session should be influenced by what the player has performed previously. One method to develop the drill complexity is to perform each part of a complex drill in isolation earlier in the progression; then, by gradually combining each component with others, a more complex drill can be performed with confidence.

Footballers love to play with the ball and will consider getting on the grass a positive step, so you should get the ball involved as early as possible. For example, if the player has a right leg injury and you do not want them to kick with the right foot at a certain stage, just get the player to use his/her left foot.

## 2.15 Communication

It is essential to have good communication between the player and staff during the rehab process. This will develop through honesty and trust. Involving the player in the process is also a useful exercise. Some players will not want to contribute much in terms of their rehab program and some will. It is therefore useful to assess the player's interest and involve the player as much or as little as they want.

Questions you ask the player during sessions can influence their response and therefore the direction in which the rehabilitation is led. For example, if you keep asking the player, *"Did you feel that?"* or *"Are you OK?"* during the session, eventually they will say they feel something. This not only can reinforce a negative presentation, but also you may then feel obliged to stop the session as you said you do not want them to feel any pain. One way to approach this is to say to the player at the start of a session *"I am NOT going to keep asking you, but if you feel uncomfortable at any time just let me know."* You may still ask the player once or twice in the session how they felt if you see something that concerns you, but it is not a good practice to ask too often. When you do ask, try to do so in a positive way, e.g., "Did that feel good?" rather than "Did that feel bad?"

## 2.16 Observation and Demonstration

With time and focus, you will become better at recognizing quality movement and also recognize when a player is not comfortable. If you are paying attention to the player's function, you can adjust what

they are doing so that they are comfortable. Conscious observation during a session is essential, particularly when you are introducing a new drill or skill.

Often you will need to demonstrate what you require the player to do, but remember that you are only really aiming to demonstrate the required movement. Players will have greater confidence in, and respect for, you if you do not try to perform skills that you are not able to do. Instead aim to demonstrate just enough for the player to understand what is required, then stop and watch the player. Remember it is their rehab not yours

## 2.17 Summary

Below are the main messages for the football doctor to consider after reading this chapter:

— You don't need to have been a great footballer to do great football rehab.
— The main goal of football rehab is to get players back to training as soon as is safely possible.
— A team of medical professionals working together will be your greatest resource.
— Good planning and being organized are essential parts of effective rehabilitation.
— Having a logical framework and philosophy of approach is important in achieving consistent results.
— You need a good diagnosis for effective rehab.
— With a system of approach that moves through logical stages of functional progression, and with an understanding of how to manipulate your rehab interventions, you should feel comfortable to rehabilitate any injury with confidence.

Developing your own philosophy of approach and your own framework of drills, protocols, and procedures will take a little time. Once you have started, however, you will appreciate the benefits of having a structure to use in your own football medicine department that is specific to *your needs and your environment*. This will be one that can continue to develop and grow as your experience does.

Appendix 0 contains an example functional football rehabilitation framework. It contains example diagrams and detailed explanations that have been designed to complement the concepts introduced in this chapter. It may be a useful resource in the development of your own rehabilitation approach and philosophy.

# Chapter 3

## Psychology

*Christopher Willis*

## 3.1 Introduction

Elite footballers, who win prestigious championships and titles, attract the attention of people all over the world, and they are considered role models for their sport and its competitions. Their extraordinary physical and psychological abilities enable them to achieve the highest level of proficiency. However, they would be unable to achieve such success without the team they have behind them, and without the professional and mental support of their teammates and the team support staff. The influence of the coaching staff and medical staff is crucial for the performance of a team and its individuals, particularly with regard to the technical, tactical, physical, and psychological aspects of performance.[1]

Players are human beings, susceptible to the pressures of everyday life, as well as those related to a high-level performance sport where their careers and their personal success depend on their achievements and those of the team surrounding them. As with all elite sports, the impact of mental preparation and the well-being of player and team performance has gained increased focus in recent years, as it has now been recognized how much psychology matters.[2]

This chapter focuses on general mental health and psychological issues relating to football, and the key instruments of a toolkit for the modern football doctor. A team physician should have a general idea which psychological factors may play a role in football, especially for peak performance. He/she should understand the psychological demands of the game, and should consider psychological factors when treating and coordinating care for injured athletes.[3]

This chapter will cover the following key areas of football psychology:
— Components of peak performance in football.
— Psychological demands of the game.
— Psychology of injuries.

## 3.2 Components of Peak Performance in Football

There are three fundamental factors related to peak performance in football:
— Culture of excellence in the football organization.
— Culture of success in a football team.
— Individual psychological components for peak performance and well-being.

Elite footballers are not simple, unidimensional beings. They are versatile and function within a highly complex social and organisational environment, which exerts major influences on them and their performance. It is helpful to incorporate all psychological topics and variables into a unifying model of psychological preparation to peak performance.[4]

### 3.2.1 Culture of Excellence in the Football Organization: A Fundamental Factor for Peak Performance

The foundation of peak performance in football is a culture of excellence, which is defined by traditions, the coaching philosophy, realistic objectives, exceptional leadership, and communications skills. A culture of excellence is by definition out of the ordinary.[5]

It directly affects the players' ability to be productive, their sense of accomplishment, and even their quality of life. Working daily at being excellent has an impact on how players interact with each other and how they handle success and failure.[2]

One important difference between winners and losers in a sport such as football is how teams handle losing.[6] Losing produces the temptation to behave in ways that make it difficult to recover fast enough psychologically, and which worsen the situation. These include for example, panicking and throwing out the game plan; scrambling for self-protection and abandoning the rest of the group; hiding facts and hoping that things will get better by themselves before anyone notices; denying that there is anything to learn or change.[6]

Striving for a culture of excellence can help prevent such behavior occurring by changing how players think about themselves, their teammates, and their team. When positive, the values, mindsets and behaviors that constitute an environment foster success, and can influence the confidence of individual players, their teammates, their coaches, and the team as a whole.[7]

### How Do You Know That a Team Lacks Trust?

There a several signs of a non-trusting team: players are afraid to speak up; members of the team keep valuable information to themselves; players do not support each other, missing participation in team discussions, etc. Anyone within a team should be looking out for these signs if they want to foster a culture of excellence. As a leader, the doctor must aim to remove debilitating fear, share information with the team, avoid micromanagement, and give up control leadership[8] (**Table 3.1**).

An environment carried by mutual respect is the basis for success. Successful football teams strive for excellence, within all their organizational structures, which includes the first team, youth teams and youth education (where applicable), and training staff, as well as the management organization, which supports the football.[10] Installing a culture of

**Table 3.1**

**Signs of culture of excellence versus signs for mistrust**

| Signs of culture of trust | Warning signs for mistrust |
|---|---|
| Open communication and information | Communication decreases |
| Convene conversations among different groups | Criticism and blame increase |
| Strive to reduce inequities and status difference | Respect decreases constant criticism |
| Communication of inspiring goals | Isolation increases—subgroups occur |
| Raise aspirations | Focus turns inward—people become self-absorbed |
| Praise those who meet high standards | Internal rivalries escalate |
| Reward initiative | Initiative decreases |
| Reinforce the positive | Negativity spreads |

*Source: Kanter 2012.*[9]

excellence does not just happen; it takes effort, but the payoffs in terms of performance and results can be priceless.

### A Team Doctor Should ...
- Be aware of signs of mistrust.
- Educate the players about the importance of a culture of excellence.
- Foster a culture of success.

### 3.2.2 Culture of Success in a Football Team

Winning in football is about teamwork. Creating an environment leading to team synergy can provide team members with a task focus (instead of focusing on results), in a socially supportive training and performance environment that cultivate success.[11]

Success in football teams requires that time and energy be devoted to building a culture that will lead to success. A culture is the expression of a team's values, attitudes, and beliefs about sport and competition. The culture is grounded in an identified sense of mission and shared goals, for instance, the goal of qualifying for final tournaments, European club competitions, or winning trophies/titles. The culture of a team, whether healthy or unhealthy, has a real impact on its individual players. For example, a team that is in constant conflict or creates a negative atmosphere will bring team members, players, and coaches alike down and this will also hurt the performances of the individual players. Conversely, a team culture built on positive energy, support, and fun will lift everyone, feel comfortable and supportive, and will be reflected in the results. The culture creates the atmosphere that permeates every aspect of a team's experience.[12]

### Build a Positive and High-Performing Sports Team Culture

However, becoming a team is an evolutionary process. Teams are constantly developing and changing in their attempts to respond to both internal and external factors. Teams move progressively through different stages of this development, and critical issues arise at each stage. Almost all teams go through four stages as they develop: these are termed forming, storming, norming and performing[13].

#### Forming

Team members familiarize themselves with other team members. Members of a team engage in social comparisons, assessing each other's strengths and weaknesses.

#### Storming

The second stage is characterized by resistance to the leader, resistance to control by the group, and interpersonal conflicts. Power struggles may occur as individuals, and the formal and informal leaders, establish their roles and status within the group. In this stage, the team members need to communicate openly.

#### Norming

In this stage, conflicts are resolved and a sense of unity formed. The players work together to reach common goals. Team roles stabilize, and a respect develops for each player's unique contribution to the team.

#### Performing

Team members will pull together to channel their energies for a team to succeed. Structural issues are resolved and interpersonal relationships have been stabilized. Roles are well defined and the players help each other to succeed; the primary goal is team success.[14]

In football, the overarching goal is to help a team to reach the performing stage as soon as possible. Team-building exercises are often done by sport psychologists to help a team through its development process. Coaches, players, and team doctors should consider the following advice to help achieve this process:

— Involve all members of the team in the team goal setting process, monitor the progress, and provide feedback related to team goals.
— Regularly assess the team's dynamics to identify at which stage of team development your team is operating.
— Schedule regular reviews of where the team is in the four-stage development process and adjust your behavior and leadership approach to suit the stage your team has reached. Incorporate team-building activities.
— Consider what needs to be done (e.g., improve communication; building interdependence and trust) to move the team effectively toward the performing stage.[15]

**A Team Doctor Should …**
— Be aware that all members of the team (not only the players) should be involved in the team goal setting process.
— Know that the team's dynamic should be regularly assessed.
— Take part in the team-building process.

### 3.2.3 Individual Psychological Components for Peak Performance and Well-Being

This model (**Fig. 3.1**) includes the personality characteristics of a footballer defined by his/her motivational orientations, values, and philosophical beliefs and his/her physical, social, psychological, and organizational environment.

Based on this model, sport psychologists focus on the working areas shown in **Table 3.2**.

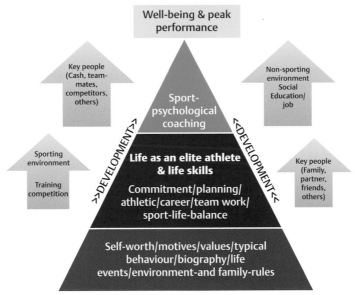

**Fig. 3.1**    A model of psychological components for peak performance and well-being. (Adapted from Hardy et al 1996.[16])

| Table 3.2 | | | |
|---|---|---|---|
| **Working areas in team culture** | | | |
| **Performance culture** | **Mental skills training** | **Individual performance** | **Teambuilding** |
| — Visions | — Performance profiling | — Self-awareness | — Building trust |
| — Values | — Goal setting | — Self-management | — Team reflection |
| — Leadership | — Concentration/attention | — Confidence | — Team identity and chemistry |
| — Communication | — Mindfulness and yoga | — Energy management | — Conflict management |
| — Talent management | — Breathing | — Social awareness | — Winning formula |
| | — Activation | — Leading yourself | |
| | — Self-talk and affirmations | — Leading others | |
| | — Visualization | — Crisis negotiation | |
| | — Rituals | | |

### 3.2.4 General Working Areas for Sport Psychologists

One possible approach for sport psychologists is to consider the following 10 beliefs when working with footballers:[17]

- The mental component plays a major role in both training and competition. Quality performances require quality training. A sports psychologist's core mission is to build quality into daily training sessions as well as during match days.
- Footballers and coaches operate with an interplay of thoughts, feelings, physiology, and actions. This interaction is crucial for performance and well-being.
- Footballers and coaches have a personality and identity (values, motives, self-esteem, and typical behaviors) that shape their lives and actions. However, many people act differently in different situations, because they are also affected by their surroundings, and adapt to different situations.
- Footballers are embedded in an environment. One cannot understand an athlete without understanding the environment and relationships between people within this environment.
- Footballers are motivated and learn better when they are allowed to think and take responsibility for their own development.
- Footballers are footballers 24 hours a day. This requires dedication and commitment.
- A football career is a progression through a series of natural phases that provide unique challenges. The transition between (or progression through) these phases is a key challenge for players, and offers the potential for crisis or growth.
- Adversity is a part of any sport. Players must learn to view adversity as a natural part of their sport and therefore develop strategies to manage and cope.
- Achieving good results is accomplished through a focus on the process, not only on the outcome.
- Mental skills should be developed in the sport environment. Therefore, the development of mental skills should be integrated into daily training sessions. The coach plays an important role in mental development.

## 3.3 Psychological Demands of the Game

Peak performance in sport is about performing at your best when it matters the most—and it matters the most in critical situations where one action can trigger major changes.[18] The pressure experienced by footballers especially at a professional level influences their playing performance. In professional football over recent years, expectations of coaches and players have increased dramatically. Fear of failure, doubts about their own abilities, dissatisfaction with their own and the team's performance, discontent with the teams philosophy of play, criticism from the manager, threats of deselection, heavy playing schedules, competition for team places, uncertain future, the media and fans, as well as the pressure to win trophies all play a part in developing high stress and anxiety levels. Even experienced players can suffer from prematch stress.[2,19] These issues can affect players in a number of harmful ways, including illness, anxiety, performance issues and over the long term - potential burnout[20] (**Fig. 3.2**).

### "Mentally Tough" Players

Sport psychologists have captured what it means to be a mentally tough player and identified 10 key factors of mental toughness in professional football:[21]

- Having total self-belief at all times that you will achieve success.
- Wanting the ball at all times (when playing well and not so well).
- Having the ability to react to situations positively.
- Having the ability to hang on and be calm under pressure.
- Knowing what it takes to get yourself out of trouble.
- Having the ability to ignore distractions and remain focused.
- Controlling emotions throughout performance.
- Having a presence that affects opponents.
- Having all aspects of life outside the game under control.
- Enjoying the pressure associated with performance.

One strong basis for creating mental toughness is that footballers have self-awareness and empathy about their own mental state. They should be able to recognize what their role is, what their emotions

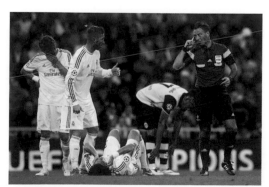

**Fig. 3.2** Even experienced players can suffer from prematch stress.

are, and how they affect their thoughts and behaviors during games.

## A Team Doctor Should ...
- Be aware of stress and anxiety levels of the players.
- Educate players about the importance of self-awareness with regard to their own mental state.
- Refer stressed players to sport psychologists.

## 3.4 Psychology of Injuries

Injuries are among the most stressful aspects of competitive sport. Serious injuries can have a variety of negative physical and psychological consequences for athletes, and may even result in the end of a season or even a career. Despite the complications of injuries, research shows that athletes who are treated with a rehabilitation program that uses psychological strategies experience a renewed perspective on sport, increased motivation, and an improved ability to cope with frustrations.[22,23,24]

Therefore, team physicians should consider psychological factors when treating and coordinating care for injured athletes. The Team Physician Consensus Statement on psychological issues proposes the following guidelines:[3]
- It is **essential** that the team physician:
  - Recognizes that psychological factors may play a role as antecedents to sports injuries.
  - Understands emotional reactions accompanying athletic injuries.
  - Understands that athletic injury programs should incorporate psychological as well as physical strategies.
  - Understands that physical clearance to return to play may not correlate to psychological readiness.
  - Identifies licensed mental health providers for athlete referrals.[25]

- It is **desirable** that the team physician:
  - Educates coaches and parents regarding the impact of major life events and stressors (death in family, divorce, life transitions) that may place athletes at greater risk for injury.
  - Educates coaches and parents regarding the effects of attitudes and behaviors that equate injury with worthlessness (e.g., no pain, no gain) that may increase stress and consequently increase injury risk.
  - Facilitates provision of psychological support services as needed.

### 3.4.1 Psychological Antecedents of Sport Injury

Psychological factors may increase the risk of sport injuries.[26] In particular, psychological stress has shown a robust association with the occurrence of injury across a variety of sports. Athletes reporting higher levels of stressful live events have consistently displayed a tendency to sustain more and more severe injuries. Common stress factors include both positive and negative events in the personal, occupational, and athletic lives of athletes. In addition to life stress, other psychological factors that contribute to either the occurrence of sport injuries or sport participation time lost due to injury include various personality factors and coping resources.

The model of stress and sport injury shown in **Fig. 3.3** represents an attempt to explain how psychological factors such as stressful events, personality, and coping resources can influence the risk of incurring sport injury. Potentially stressful situations are thought to affect the injury vulnerability through a process in which interpretations of the situations influence, and are influenced by, physiological and attentional changes.

The model underscores the importance of getting to know your players. It is important for team

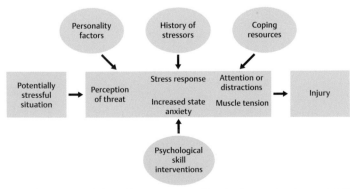

**Fig. 3.3** A model of stress and sport injury. (Adapted from Brewer 2009[26] and Williams and Andersen 1998.[27])

physicians to be mindful observers of players entrusted in their care, taking note of individual dispositions (general patterns of behavior), so as to be in a better position to determine how a player's personality may heighten or reduce injury risk as stress ebbs and flows over the season."[28]

### 3.4.2 Injury Rehabilitation

The occurrence of an injury can have both a physical and psychological effect on the player. Feltz contents that a sports injury has three psychological effects on an athlete:[29] (1) emotional trauma of the injury, (2) psychological factors associated with rehabilitation and recovery; and (3) the psychological impact of the injury on the athlete's future.[30]

The injured athlete's experience is a complex interrelationship of thoughts, feelings, and behaviors. Understanding the process by which athletes psychologically respond to injuries is of importance. It would be helpful for team doctors to be mindful that each individual's experience is unique; consequently, no single theory or model can be applied indiscriminately.[30]

Team physicians can exert a positive influence on athletes by developing a positive rapport and by simply communicating effectively. Listening to athletes, explaining rehabilitation activities clearly, avoiding jargon and overly technical terminology, controlling nonverbal behavior, and recognizing athletes' needs for informational as well as socioemotional communication are some ways that sport medicine professionals can interact with athletes to create an environment that is conducive to adherence to rehabilitation.[31] In these situations, psychological interventions can offer significant benefits to an athlete's rehabilitation in terms of having more information and understanding of rehabilitation, having an increased sense of responsibility and control over their recoveries, and having their physical and psychological needs met in an organized and comprehensive manner.[32]

Research suggests that maintaining a positive attitude, social support, and using mental skills (such as educational interventions, goal setting, and imagery) are related to a shorter rehabilitation. In fact, when Ievleva and Orlick compared slow and fast healers, they found that the fast healers[33,34]
- Took personal responsibility for healing.
- Had high desire and determination.
- Had more social support.
- Maintained a positive attitude.
- Used creative visualization.
- Were less fearful of reinjury upon return to full participation.[33]

### 3.4.3 Educational Interventions

Education can make athletes aware of their situation.[35] Research has shown that athletes who do not have a clear vision of the rehabilitation process experience negative emotions and demotivation.[36] That is why it is important to intervene in the early stages of the rehabilitation.[37] In this phase, it is important that doctors provide an anatomical description of the injury and a timetable of the recovery. Afterward, it is necessary that players know how the recovery process involves muscle soreness and stasis, and that not only the injury, but also the rehabilitation produces pain.[34] Players should learn to not use painkillers excessively and to recognize injury pains, which are negative symptoms, and rehabilitation pains, which are positive symptoms.[34,38] Players should also be prepared with regards to their oncoming emotions, such as frustration, anger, or mood swings. It is also necessary that they are conscious of their role in the rehabilitation programme, and the importance of their compliance with the medical staff. Education restrains the emotions and attitudes typical of denial and distress phases, such as anxiety, depression, resistances, and loss of self-confidence. Consequently, their duration reduces, anticipating a determined coping attitude[34,37] (**Fig. 3.4**).

### 3.4.4 Goal Setting[39]

Research on the goal setting process during sport injury rehabilitation has shown that it has multiple benefits to the athlete. For example, setting goals during rehabilitation has been found to have a positive effect on the athlete's physiological and psychological healing.[39,41] It also appears that goal setting has a positive impact on athletes' attitude, successful acceptance of the injury, overall confidence in the injury recovery, as well as adherence to the rehabilitation programme.[42,43]

According to Taylor and Taylor,[40] the process for goal setting should begin with a conversation between the rehabilitation professionals and the athlete, in

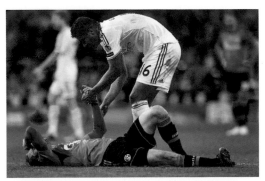

**Fig. 3.4** Players should be prepared with regard to their oncoming emotions, such as frustration, anger, or mood swings.

**3**

which critical physical aspects of rehabilitation are discussed and explained. This should then be followed by clear goal setting for each of the components of physical recovery, including range of motion, strength, stability, stamina, flexibility, and any other relevant physical parameters. Psychological goals should be discussed in a similar manner.[39] Finally, the set goals need to be revised and assessed with the sport medicine professionals on a regular basis in order for them to be effective.[40,44]

### 3.4.5 Imagery

Mental imagery may be the most powerful mental training tool that players can have at their disposal.[45] Many athletes appreciate the usefulness of mental imagery in enhancing sport performance.[39,46] Imagery can be described as an activity which involves creating a clear mental picture of sporting situations, which can mean the venue, the performance, the conditions, the people, and the emotions and feelings. When applied to sport injury rehabilitation in football, injury can be seen as an activity in which the player can create images of the healing process, the injured body part fully healed and restored to normal levels of functioning, the rehabilitation exercises, dealing with pain, and any emotions associated with the injury and recovery process.[39]

Rehabilitation imagery can prepare athletes for the challenges of rehabilitation including surgery, pain, setbacks, and a return to sport. Athletes can imagine feeling calm and relaxed before surgery, being motivated and intense during physical therapy exercises, feeling confident when returning to the athletic arena and performing aggressively with the recovered body part during competition. Rehabilitation imagery is a skill that develops with practice.[45]

Walsh[47] compiled the existing information and listed four main types of imagery beneficial to sport injury rehabilitation:

- Healing imagery (i.e., visualizing and feeling the injured body part healing).
- Pain management imagery (i.e., assisting the athlete to cope with pain associated with the injury).
- Rehabilitation process imagery (i.e., assisting in dealing with challenges that athletes may encounter during the rehabilitation program).
- Performance imagery (i.e., practicing physical skills and imagining oneself performing successfully and injury free).[39,47]

Richardson and Latuda[48] proposed a four-step programme showing how imagery could be integrated into injury rehabilitation.[39,47] Arvinen-Barrow et al[39] modified this program by including an additional step:

- Imagery should be introduced by the team physician to the injured player with the intention of

educating him/her about the practical application and potential benefits which could be derived from its incorporation into injury rehabilitation.[39]
- The player's imagery ability needs to be informally assessed (ideally by a sport psychologist). The information obtained from this assessment can then be used in the development of an imagery programme to be incorporated into the athlete's injury rehabilitation.[39]
- The player needs to be assisted in the development of basic imagery skills[39] (ideally by a sport psychologist).
- Players need to commit to practicing the use of the skill until it becomes automatic.
- Once the player has put in the necessary time practicing their use of imagery, it can be incorporated into their injury rehabilitation programme, making sure to keep the process as simple and concise as possible.[39]

Psychological interventions are most successful if used as part of a wider rehabilitation programme.[49] By attending to the psychological needs of an injured player, the doctor and other staff are treating the whole person, and not just the injury, and thus offering a more holistic approach to recovery.[49] Team doctors should take a leading role in cultivating this multidisciplinary approach to rehabilitation.[50]

## References

[1] Horn S. Coaching effectiveness in the sport domain. In: Horn S. eds. Advances in Sport Psychology. Champaign, IL: Human Kinetics; 2008:239–267

[2] Nesti M. Psychology in football. New York, NY: Routledge; 2010

[3] American, College of Sports Medicine, American Academy of Family Physicians, American Academy of Orthopaedic Surgeons, American Medical Society for Sports Medicine, American Orthopaedic Society for Sports Medicine, American Osteopathic Academy of Sports Medicine. Psychological issues related to injury in athletes and the team physician: a consensus statement. Med Sci Sports Exerc. 2006; 38(11):2030–2034

[4] Hardy L, Jones G, Gould D. Understanding Psychological Preparation for Sport. West Sussex, UK: Wiley-Blackwell; 1996:239–240

[5] http://www.sparkss.com/media/10709/Culture_Article-bt-Effective-Environments.pdf. Accessed January 18, 2015

[6] Kanter RM. Cultivate a culture of confidence. Harvard Business Review. April 2011. https://hbr.org/2011/04/column-cultivate-a-culture-of-confidence. Accessed January 18, 2015

[7] Meehan P, Rigby D, Rogers P. Creating and sustaining a winning culture. Harvard Business Review. February 2008. https://hbr.org/2008/02/creating-and-sustaining-a-winn-1. Accessed January 18, 2015

[8] Pixton P. (2008). Creating a culture of trust. http://www.accelinnova.com/docs/trustp2.doc. Accessed January 18, 2015

[9] Kanter RM. Fight the nine symptoms of corporate decline. Harvard Business Review. December 2012. https://hbr.org/2012/12/fight-the-nine-symptoms-of-cor. Accessed January 18, 2015

[10] Waal A. The high performance soccer club. http://www.talkinbusiness.nl/2014/05/the-high-performance-soccer-club. Accessed January 18, 2015

[11] Vernacchia RA. Working with individual team sports: the psychology of track and field. In: Lidor R, Henschen KP, eds. The Psychology of Team Sports. Morgantown, WV: Fitness Information Technology; 2009:257

[12] Taylor J, Build a Positive and High Performing Sports Team Culture. Retrieved from http://www.huffingtonpost.com/dr-jim-taylor/build-a-positive-and-high_b_3659341.html. Accessed January 18, 2015

[13] Weinberg S, Gould D. Foundations of Sport & Exercise Psychology. 3rd ed. Champaign, IL: Human Kinetics; 2003:157–158

[14] Weinberg S, Gould D. Foundations of Sport & Exercise Psychology. 3rd ed. Champaign: Human Kinetics; 2003

[15] Carron AV, Burke SM, Shapcott KM. Enhancing team effectiveness. In: Brewer BW, ed. Sport Psychology. West Sussex, UK: Wiley-Blackwell; 2009:64–74

[16] Hardy L, Jones G, Gould D. Understanding Psychological Preparation for Sport. West Sussex, UK: Wiley-Blackwell; 1996:240

[17] Henriksen K, Diment G, Hansen J. Professional philosophy: inside the delivery of sport psychology service at Team Denmark. Sport Sci Rev (Singap). 2011; 20(1–2):5–21

[18] Csoka, L. Peak Performance Mental Skills Workbook. Charlotte, NC: Apex Performance; 2013:2

[19] Wieser R, Thiel H. A survey of "mental hardiness" and "mental toughness" in professional male football players. Chiropr Man Therap. 2014; 22:17

[20] Williams MA. Science and Soccer. Developing Elite Performers. 3rd ed. London: Routledge; 2013

[21] Thelwell R, Weston N, Greenlees I. Defining and understanding mental toughness within soccer. J Appl Sport Psychol. 2005; 17(4):326–332

[22] Galli N. Thriving through sport injury. http://www.appliedsportpsych.org/resource-center/injury-rehabilitation/thriving-through-sport-injury. Accessed January 18, 2015

[23] Podlog L, Eklund RC. A longitudinal investigation of competitive athletes' return to sport following serious injury. J Appl Sport Psychol. 2006; 18(1):44–68

[24] Brown C. Injuries: the psychology of recovery and rehab. In: Murphy S, ed. The Sport Psych Handbook. Champaign, IL: Human Kinetics; 2005:12

[25] http://www.aafp.org/dam/AAFP/documents/patient_care/fitness/ACSMissuesrelatedtoinjury.pdf. Accessed December 1, 2016

[26] Brewer BW. Injury prevention and rehabilitation. In: Brewer B, ed. Sport Psychology. West Sussex, UK: Wiley-Blackwell; 2009:75–77

[27] Williams JM, Andersen MB. Psychosocial antecedents of sport injury: review and critique of the stress and injury model. J Appl Sport Psychol. 1998; 10:5–25

[28] Appaneal RN, Habif S. Psychological antecedents to sport injury. In: Arvinen-Barrow M, Walker N, eds. The Psychology of Sport injury and Rehabilitation. London: Routledge; 2013

[29] Feltz DL. The psychology of sport injuries. In: Vinger PF, Hoerner EF, eds. Sports Injuries: The Unthwarted Epidemic. 2nd ed. Littleton, MA: PSG Publishing; 1986:336–344

[30] Bacon VL. Psychological factors in rehabilitation. In: Andrews JR, Harrelson G, Wilk K, eds. Physical Rehabilitation of the Injured Athlete. Philadelphia, PA: Elsevier; 2012:5

[31] Granquist MD, Brewer BW. Psychological aspects of rehabilitation adherence. In: Arvinen-Barrow M, Walker N, eds. The Psychology of Sport injury and Rehabilitation. London: Routledge; 2013:40–54

[32] Heil J. Psychology of Sport Injury. Champaign: Human Kinetics; 1993

[33] Dworsky D, Krane V. (2014) Using the Mind to Hal the Body: Imagery for Injury Rehabilitation. Association for Applied Sport Psychology. http://appliedsportpsych.org/resource-center/injury-rehabilitation/using-the-mind-to-heal-the-body-imagery-for-injury-rehabilitation

[34] Ievleva L, Orlick T. Mental paths to enhanced recovery from a sports injury. In: Pargman D, ed. Psychological basis of Sport Injuries. 2nd ed. Morgantown, WV: Fitness Information Technology; 1999

[35] Santi G, Pietrantoni L. Psychology of sport injury rehabilitation: a review of models and interventions. J Hum Sport Exerc. 2013; 8 (4):1029–1044

[36] Francis SR, Andersen MB, Maley P. Physiotherapists' and male professional athletes' views on psychological skills for rehabilitation. J Sci Med Sport. 2000; 3(1):17–29

[37] O'Connor E, Heil J, Harmer P, Zimmerman I. Injury. In: Taylor J, Wilson G, eds. Applying Sport Psychology. Champaign, IL: Human Kinetics; 2005:187–206

[38] Taylor J, Taylor S. Pain education and management in the rehabilitation from sports injury. Sport Psychologist. 1998; 12(1):68–88

[39] Arvinen-Barrow M, Clement D, Hemmings B. Psychological aspects of rehabilitation adherence. In: Arvinen-Barrow M, Walker N, eds. The Psychology of Sport injury and Rehabilitation. London: Routledge; 2013

[40] Taylor J, Taylor S. Psychological Approaches to Sports Injury Rehabilitation. Gaithersburg, MD: Aspen; 1997

[41] Ievleva L, Orlick T. Mental links to enhanced healing: An exploratory study. Sport Psychol. 1991; 5(1):25–40

[42] Arvinen-Barrow M, Hemmings B. Goal setting in sport injury rehabilitation. In: Arvinen-Barrow M, Walker N, eds. The Psychology of Sport injury and Rehabilitation. London: Routledge; 2013:56–70

[43] Armatas V, Chondrou E, Yiannakos A, Galazoulas C, Velkopoulos C. Psycholopgical aspects of rehabilitation following serious athletic injuries with special reference to goal setting: a review study. Physical Training, January. In: Arvinen-Barrow M, Walker N, eds. The Psychology of Sport injury and Rehabilitation. London: Routledge; 2007

[44] Gould D. Goal setting for peak performance. In: Williams J, ed. Applied Sport Psychology: Personal Growth to Peak Performance. Palo Alto, CA: Mayfield; 1986:133–148

[45] Connor O, Heil J, Harmer P. Injury. In: Taylor J, Wilson G, eds. Applying Sport Psychology: Four Perspectives. Champaign: Human Kinetics; 2005:187–206

[46] Hall CR. Imagery in sport and exercise. In: Singer R, Hausenblas H, Janelle C, eds. Handbook of Sport Psychology. New York: Wiley; 2001:529–549

[47] Walsh M. Injury rehabilitation and imagery. In: Morris IT, Spittle M, Watt AP, eds. Imagery in Sport. Champaign, IL: Human Kinetics; 2005:267–284

[48] Richardson PA, Latuda LM. Therapeutic imagery and athletic injuries. J Athl Train. 1995; 30(1):10–12

[49] Arvinen-Barrow M, Walker N. Introduction to the psychology of sport injuries. In: Arvinen-Barrow M, Walker N, eds. The Psychology of Sport injury and Rehabilitation. London: Routledge; 2013:2–5

[50] Clement D, Arvinen-Barrow M. Sport medicine team influences in psychological rehabilitation. In: Arvinen-Barrow M, Walker N, eds. The Psychology of Sport injury and Rehabilitation. London: Routledge; 2013:171–184

# Chapter 4

## Football Nutrition

*Ronald J. Maughan*

## 4.1 Nutrition Goals and Eating Strategies

Football competitions are structured to ensure that the outcome is always in doubt. Whenever highly talented, motivated, and well-trained players play, the margin between victory and defeat is small. Attention to detail can make that vital difference. Nutrition and hydration are not major factors in performance compared with talent, skill, and fitness, but poor food choices will prevent the talented player from being able to fully demonstrate their skills. What we eat and how much we eat affect every aspect of our performance, and the foods that we choose in both training and competition will affect how well we train and play.

All players need to be aware of their personal nutritional goals and of how they can select an eating strategy to meet those goals. There are some general principles that apply to every player, but every player is different, and there is no single diet that meets the needs of all players at all times. Individual needs also change across the season and players must be flexible to accommodate this.

Each player should be aware of his or her nutritional goals, which means having some idea of the following:

- The amounts of energy, carbohydrate, protein, and water that are needed on a daily basis.
- How this intake should be distributed over the day in relation to training and match play.
- How needs vary across the season and from day to day.

More important than knowing goals in terms of nutrients is to know what foods can be chosen to meet these needs and which combinations of foods can help ensure an adequate intake of vitamins, minerals, and the various other components that contribute to health and performance.

### 4.1.1 Nutritional Assessment

As part of the preseason medical screening of players, it might be useful to include a nutritional assessment. This should include a review of the player's diet to assess whether appropriate food choices are being made. Biochemical screening for nutrient adequacy is favored by some but not by all, and there is no uniform agreement on interpretation of results of laboratory analyses. Where there is reason to suggest that a problem might exist (such as iron deficiency in a vegetarian player who reports unusual levels of fatigue) and where there is a good diagnostic test, such screening would seem appropriate. Body mass and body fat content should also be assessed and included in the player's medical records. Expert input should be sought for the implementation and interpretation of these tests (**Fig. 4.1**).

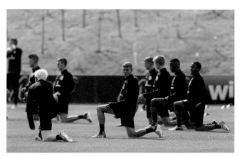

**Fig. 4.1**  The aim of training, whether for strength, speed, or stamina, is to induce changes in the structure and function of muscle that will lead to performance improvements.

## 4.2 Energy and Macronutrients for Training and Match Play

Diet may have its biggest impact on training, and a good diet will help support consistent intensive training while limiting the risks of illness or injury. The aim of training, whether for strength, speed, or stamina, is to induce changes in the structure and function of muscle that will lead to performance improvements. This requires breakdown of some proteins in the muscle and an increased rate of synthesis of others: creating the right nutrient, metabolic, and hormonal environment can promote that process. Good food choices can therefore promote the adaptations to the training stimulus that take place in the muscle during and after each training session.

### 4.2.1 Energy and Body Fat

Getting the right amount of energy to stay healthy and to perform well is key. If the energy intake is too high and body fat increases: too little and performance falls, injuries are more likely to occur, and illness often results. The average young male expends about 2,500 kcal (10 MJ) per day. To this must be added the energy cost of training, and the typical energy cost of a hard training session in top professional players is about 1,500 kcal (6 MJ). Female players, on average, have a lower body mass and train at a lower intensity, so the energy demands are correspondingly lower. The variation between individuals is large, though, further emphasizing the need to individualize advice. Daily energy demand may reach 5,000 kcal (20 MJ) on a few days in preseason training for some players. The usual daily energy expenditure is much less than this for most days of the year, though, and players should be aware of the need to balance the amount they eat with the amount of energy they expend.

If energy intake is too high, body fat levels will increase, but if it is too low, recovery will be incomplete and there is a risk of cumulative fatigue. The training load and other activities outside training will set the player's energy budget: a high energy intake usually means a high intake of all essential nutrients and gives greater flexibility in food choices. During periods of low energy intake (the off-season, during injury, or when trying to lose weight), the energy budget will be lower and more care is needed in food choices to ensure an adequate consumption of all nutrients.

The energy demand is influenced by many different factors, so it is difficult to make recommendations for individuals without assessing activity patterns. In practice, it is almost impossible to prescribe energy intake from estimates of energy expenditure: the errors of the estimates are simply too large to be reliable. It is usually better to look at body weight and body composition: if weight is stable and body fat content is at a reasonable level, energy intake must be close to energy expenditure. This requires an estimate of body fat, which can be simply achieved with a number of different methods. It should be recognized, though, that there is no single value of body fat content that is appropriate for all individuals. Some players will perform at their best with values that are higher than the average.

Although there is less focus on body image issues in football than in some other sports, all support staff should be alert to the fact that some players may be overconcerned with their physique and appearance. Some will spend too much time in the gym and some will starve themselves in an attempt to meet their ideal body image. Where this compromises performance or health, staff must intervene. For female players, this may be accompanied by irregular or absent menstruation: to avoid irreversible skeletal damage, any female player with disruption of normal menstrual function should be investigated without delay. For male players, the warning signs may be less obvious but are nonetheless real.

If there is a need to reduce body fat, this is usually apparent at the start of preseason, and a plan can be put in place to achieve the necessary changes to diet and training to achieve the desired physique without affecting playing performance. This requires coordinated input from all support staff, including the nutritionist, doctor, and strength and conditioning staff. It is possible with careful attention to diet and training to achieve a reduction in body fat levels while maintaining or even increasing lean mass. Some players are known to use weight loss supplements and "fat burners" to help them achieve their target weight, but this is to be strongly discouraged. Most of these supplements do not work and those that do carry serious health risks, including especially liver damage. Some herbal weight loss products have been shown to contain anorectic agents

and stimulants that are not declared on the label but that will result in a positive doping result. This is discussed in more detail in Chapter 6.

## 4.2.2 Carbohydrate

Carbohydrate supplies the muscles and brain with the fuels they need to meet the demands of training and competition. A high carbohydrate intake is essential during periods of hard training, but less is needed for most of the season and in the off-season. Players must be aware of what foods they should choose to meet their carbohydrate needs, how much should be eaten, and when these foods should be eaten (**Fig. 4.2**).

Carbohydrate is an important fuel for high-intensity exercise, but the body can only store enough to last for 1 day of hard training. Each player's everyday eating and drinking plan therefore needs to provide enough carbohydrate to fuel their training program and to optimize the recovery of muscle glycogen stores between workouts. General recommendations can be provided for carbohydrate intake, based on the player's body size and the demands of their training program, but actual needs are specific to the individual, and must be fine-tuned to take account of the total energy needs and specific training goals. It is important to get feedback from performance in training and match play to assess whether there is a problem with fuel availability. An inadequate carbohydrate intake will lead to early fatigue.

There is a sound body of evidence to suggest that carbohydrate intake strategies which maintain high carbohydrate availability during exercise and prevent carbohydrate depletion are associated with enhanced endurance and performance during many types of sporting activities. These strategies include ensuring high levels of muscle and liver glycogen prior to exercise, the intake of a carbohydrate-rich meal in the hours before training or match play, the intake of carbohydrate during games, and the intake

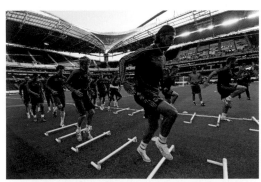

**Fig. 4.2** It is important to get feedback from performance in training and match play to assess whether there is a problem with fuel availability.

of carbohydrate in the recovery period between two bouts of carbohydrate-demanding exercise.

The primary source of carbohydrate comes from the diet, and sugar- and starch-rich foods can contribute to energy and fuel needs as well as providing other useful nutrients for health and performance. However, special sports products containing substantial amounts of carbohydrate provide a valuable nutrition aid in some situations. The advantages or value of these products include taste appeal, provision of a known amount of carbohydrate to meet a specific sports nutrition goal, simultaneous provision of other important nutrients for sports nutrition goals, and gastrointestinal characteristics promoting quick digestion and absorption. Other benefits relate to characteristics that make the products practical to consume around exercise sessions (low bulk, conveniently packaged) or in the athlete's lifestyle (portable, nonperishable, minimal preparation). When these sports products are used by an athlete to meet the sports nutrition situations outlined above, they are likely to enhance performance, though perhaps no more so than could be achieved with carefully selected normal foods. The performance benefits achieved by addressing a situation that would otherwise result in low carbohydrate availability are robust, ranking carbohydrate supplements among the nutritional performance enhancers with the strongest evidence base in sports nutrition.

When the period between training sessions is less than about 8 hours (as in twice daily preseason training for elite players), carbohydrate intake, in the form of solids or liquids, should start as soon as practicable after the first session to maximize the effective recovery time. There may be some advantages in meeting carbohydrate targets through a series of snacks during the early recovery phase. Consuming foods with a high glycemic index (i.e., those that result in rapid and large elevations of the blood glucose concentration) may be useful at this time. Examples of carbohydrate foods with moderate-high glycemic index include the following:

— Most breakfast cereals.
— Most forms of rice.
— White and brown breads.
— Sports drinks and soft drinks.
— Sugar, jam, and honey.
— Potatoes.
— Tropical fruits and juices.

During longer recovery periods (24 hours), the pattern and timing of carbohydrate-rich meals and snacks do not appear to be critical, and can be organized according to what is practical and comfortable for each player. There is no difference in glycogen synthesis when carbohydrate is consumed in liquid form or as solid foods, even though there may be some differences in the rates of digestion and absorption. Given the amount of carbohydrate to be consumed, high carbohydrates foods will need to be spread out over the full 24 hours.

It is valuable to choose nutrient-rich carbohydrates and to add other foods to recovery meals and snacks to provide protein and other nutrients. These nutrients may assist in other recovery processes, and in the case of protein, may promote additional glycogen recovery when carbohydrate intake is below targets or when frequent snacking is not possible. Adequate energy intake is also important for optimal glycogen recovery, but the restrained eating practices of some players, particularly females, can make it difficult to meet carbohydrate intake targets and to optimize glycogen storage from this intake. Examples of nutrient-rich carbohydrate foods and meal combinations include the following:

— Breakfast cereal with milk.
— Flavored yoghurt.
— Fruit smoothie or liquid meal supplement.
— Sandwich with meat and salad filling.
— Stir fry with rice or noodles.
— Meat, potatoes, and vegetables.
— Vegetable curry and bread.

Similar strategies apply to recovery after games. This can be especially challenging after matches that finish late in the evening, with further complications if there is a homeward journey beginning immediately after the match. Neglecting an adequate carbohydrate intake after the game will delay recovery and it is important that some carbohydrate is consumed before setting off on the journey home and before going to bed.

Low-carbohydrate diets have been promoted for athletes in recent years without clear evidence of benefits to performance. Training with restricted carbohydrate availability may enhance the capacity for fat oxidation during exercise, but it seems that a performance benefit does not necessarily result, at least under the protocols used in the currently available literature in which 50 to 100% of training sessions have been undertaken in this manner. When muscle glycogen stores are low, there may be some impairment of performance in high-intensity sprints, and these are often the most crucial movements during a game. There must also be a concern that training or playing with low carbohydrate availability may increase the risk of injury and illness. The evidence for the former is limited, but there are some suggestions of increased injury rates in athletes training and competing with low muscle glycogen levels.

### 4.2.3 Protein

The aim of training is to improve performance and protein plays a key role in the adaptations that take place in response to training. Amino acids from proteins are the building blocks for the manufacture of new tissue, including muscle, and the repair of old or damaged tissue. They are also the structural precursors for hormones and enzymes that regulate metabolism and other body functions. Protein provides only a small source of fuel for the exercising muscle, but any protein consumed in excess of the amount that can be used immediately will be used as a fuel for energy supply. Because of this, there is no advantage in eating more protein than is necessary. High-protein diets are not usually harmful, but eating too much protein will displace carbohydrate from the diet.

The average sedentary person needs about 0.6 g of protein per kilogram body mass per day (g/kg/d). To ensure that everyone gets enough, a safety margin is added to the recommendations, and a daily intake of about 0.8 to 0.9 g/kg is usually recommended. It has long been recognized that regular hard exercise results in an increased requirement for dietary protein, but there has been much disagreement over the amount that is appropriate. Some scientists have suggested that combined endurance and resistance-training exercise will increase daily protein needs up to a maximum of 1.2 to 1.6 g/kg, but some recommend even higher amounts.

The debate over the precise protein needs of players is largely unnecessary. Dietary surveys show that most players who eat enough to meet their energy needs already consume diets that provide protein intakes above 1.2 to 1.6 g/kg/d, even without the use of protein supplements. Therefore, most players do not need to be encouraged or educated to increase their protein intakes. Rather, anyone who consumes adequate energy intake from a variety of nutrient-rich foods should be confident of meeting their protein needs, including any increases that could arise from high-level training. Players most at risk of failing to meet their protein needs are those who severely restrict their energy intake for long periods or who eat a monotonous diet. An adequate energy intake is also important in promoting protein balance or increasing protein retention.

Some resistance-trained athletes and body builders consume very large amounts of protein (as much as 3–4 g/kg/d) and players who spend time in the gym will invariably pick up some of these ideas, but there is no evidence that such dietary patterns enhance the response to training or increase the gains in muscle mass and strength. While such diets are not necessarily harmful, they are expensive in purely financial terms (this is not an issue for the elite player, but their practices will be followed by those with more limited financial means) and can result in players failing to meet other nutritional goals, such as providing the fuel needed to optimize training and performance. A small excess of protein is unlikely to be harmful for healthy individuals, but too much protein may not leave enough room for carbohydrate and essential fats within the player's energy budget. High-protein diets can also become high-fat diets if players are not careful to choose lean protein options.

### 4.2.4 Timing of Intake

New research within the last decade or so shows that the timing of intake of protein as well as the total amount that is consumed will have important consequences for net protein synthesis. Regular intake at intervals over the day also seems to be important in maximizing responses. Recent studies have focused on the acute response to workouts of both endurance and resistance training. Enhanced protein balance is a desirable goal of the recovery phase to overturn the increased rates of protein breakdown that normally occur during exercise, and to promote muscle growth, repair, and adaptation following the exercise stimulus. These studies have found that the intake of small amounts (about 20–25 g) of high-quality protein enhances protein synthesis during the recovery period. Further work is required to fine-tune guidelines for the optimum amount, type, and timing of intake of these nutrients and to confirm that these eating strategies lead to an enhancement of the goals of training. It should be remembered also that the focus on match day should be entirely on performance: on other days, nutrition strategies are geared toward the long-term goals.

In the light of this information, it appears sensible to focus on the total balance of the diet and the timing of protein–carbohydrate meals and snacks in relation to training, rather than on high-protein intakes per se. Such a combination of protein and carbohydrate can look after refueling and protein recovery needs. Special sports foods such as sports bars and liquid meal supplements can provide a compact and convenient way to consume carbohydrate and protein when everyday foods are unavailable or are too bulky and impractical to consume. However, the additional cost of these products and the fact that most contain only a limited range of nutrients must be taken into account. There is little justification for using very expensive protein-only powders or amino acid supplements as everyday foods are likely to be just as effective, and perhaps even better because of the wide range of additional nutrients they contain.

Each of the following food choices will provide 10 g of high-quality protein:

— Two small eggs.
— Cow's milk: 300 mL.
— Skim milk powder: 20 g.
— cheese: 30 g.
— Yoghurt: 200 g.
— Meat, fish, or chicken: 35 to 50 g.
— Fruit smoothie or liquid meal supplement: 150 mL.

Well-chosen vegetarian diets can easily meet protein needs. Each of the following vegetarian choices will provide 10 g of high-quality protein:

— Four slices of bread.
— Breakfast cereal: 90 g.
— Two cups of cooked pasta or three cups of rice.
— soy milk: 400 mL.
— Nuts or seeds: 60 g.
— Tofu or soy meat: 120 g.
— Legumes or lentils: 150 g.

Players restricting energy intake—whether to achieve weight loss or to prevent weight gain during periods of reduced training (e.g., after injury)—may need to be more careful in choosing protein-rich foods because total food intake will be less. There is some evidence that a higher-than-normal protein intake may be desirable to maintain muscle mass when energy intake is low.

## 4.3 Hydration Strategies

When players work hard, they lose sweat—in a game on a hot day, sweat losses may reach 3 L in some players, though they are more typically about 1 to 2 L in a typical training session or match. Female players generally sweat less than their male counterparts, but as in so many areas of human nutrition, there is an enormous interindividual variability, and some players will lose very little sweat. Every player's hydration needs are different and will vary with the weather over the season. Just as general training and competition strategies should be tailored for individual athletes in accordance with their unique needs and preferences, so should their drinking and eating choices during exercise. Players, coaches, and trainers should "fine-tune" these recommendations to identify their own optimum formula.

### 4.3.1 How Much and When to Drink

Players should aim to limit dehydration during training and matches by drinking water or a sports drink, but there are many occasions where it may not be necessary or helpful to drink at all. During training, the coach or manager should organize drink breaks according to the weather and intensity of the session. Obvious opportunities to drink during a match include warm-up and at half time, but stoppages for injury can also be used if necessary, subject to the agreement of the referee.

Training allows opportunities for players to get a feel for their sweat rates and fluid needs so that drink practices can be adjusted accordingly. It is not necessary to drink enough to match sweat loss, but the amount of dehydration should normally be limited to a loss of less than about 2% of body weight (i.e., 1.5 kg for a 75-kg person). Some may choose to drink according to the dictates of thirst, but there are many distractions during a game and awareness of thirst does not always coincide with drinking opportunities.

Dehydration, if sufficiently severe, will impair both physical and mental performance, and these effects are greater in warm environments, so drinking practices in these conditions should be upgraded to reduce the overall fluid deficit. This may include drinking at the sideline when match play is interrupted, or having extra drink breaks during training sessions. There should never be a need to drink more than the sweat loss so that weight is gained during exercise. This will not help performance and is likely to cause discomfort (**Fig. 4.3**).

Depletion of fuel stores can be an issue for football matches, and high-carbohydrate strategies—fuelling up for the game and consuming extra carbohydrate during the match—have been shown to enhance performance, or at least distance covered and amount of distance covered at sprinting speed. Better intake of fluid and fuel during a game may not only keep players running further and faster in the second half of a match, but also help maintain skills and judgment when players would otherwise become fatigued. Games are often won and lost in the last minutes of the match, and fatigued players are at increased risk of injury. The use of commercial sports drinks with a carbohydrate content of about 4 to 8% (4–8 g/100 mL) allows carbohydrate and fluid needs to be met simultaneously in most events. The intake of

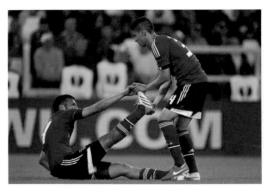

**Fig. 4.3**   Dehydration, if sufficiently severe, will impair both physical and mental performance.

carbohydrate that is generally associated with performance benefits is approximately 20 to 60 g/h.

For most players, some sodium might usefully be included in fluids consumed during matches or in training sessions lasting longer than 1 hour. There is some evidence, largely anecdotal, that players who lose a lot of salt may be more prone to muscle cramps. You can recognize those whose sweat has a high salt content by the salt rings on their clothes at the end of a hard session on a hot day. Adding a little extra salt to food and drinks and using the higher sodium version of sports drinks may reduce the risk of cramping for these players, but probably does not benefit all players (**Fig. 4.4**).

## 4.3.2 Caffeine

Caffeine is present in many commonly available drinks (tea, coffee, cola, etc.) and sports foods (e.g., gels, some sports drinks) and can enhance performance in some situations. This benefit can be obtained with the relatively small doses of caffeine that are commonly consumed by people of various cultures (e.g., about 2–3 mg/kg bodyweight as found in 1–2 cups of brewed coffee or 750–1,500 mL of a cola beverage). Caffeine is a diuretic agent, but these amounts will not compromise fluid balance. Strategic use of caffeine, which is not on the World Anti-Doping Agency (WADA) prohibited list (though its use is monitored during competition), may therefore be helpful to some, but perhaps not all, players.

## 4.3.3 How to Estimate Sweating Rate

- Measure body weight (kg) both before and after at least 1 hour of exercise under conditions similar to competition or a hard practice.
- Measure body weight wearing minimal clothing and while bare footed. Towel dry after exercise and obtain body weight as soon as is practical after exercise (e.g., less than 10 min).

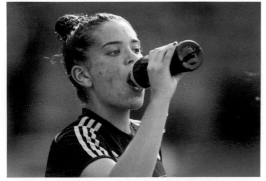

**Fig. 4.4** For most players, some sodium might usefully be included in fluids consumed during matches or in training sessions lasting longer than 1 hour.

- Note volume of fluid consumed during exercise (L).
- Sweat loss (L) = Body weight before exercise (kg) – Body weight after exercise (kg) + fluid consumed during exercise (L).
- To convert to a sweat rate per hour, divide by the exercise time in minutes and multiply by 60.

> **NOTE:**
>
> 2.2 lb equals 1.0 kg and converts to a volume of 1.0 L or 1,000 mL or 34 oz of water.

## 4.3.4 Rehydration after Exercise

Recovery after exercise is part of the preparation for the next exercise session, and replacement of sweat losses is an essential part of this process. Both water and salts lost in sweat must be replaced. After a few sessions of weighing themselves before and after training or matches, players should have a good idea of their typical sweat losses in different environmental conditions. They should aim to drink about 1.2 to 1.5 L of fluid for each kilogram of weight lost in training or matches. Drinks should contain sodium (the main salt lost in sweat) if no food is eaten at this time, but most meals will contain adequate amounts of salt. Sports drinks that contain electrolytes can be helpful, though the amounts they contain are generally very small, but many foods can also supply the salt that is needed. A little extra salt may be added to meals when sweat losses are high, but salt tablets should be used with caution.

## 4.3.5 Alcohol

Alcohol is not an essential component of a diet, and it is a personal choice whether an adult player consumes alcohol at all. However, it is important to recognize that there is no evidence of impairments to health and performance when alcohol is used sensibly.

As well as providing a source of energy, alcohol (ethanol) acts as a drug that has metabolic, cardiovascular, thermoregulatory, and neuromuscular actions that may affect exercise performance. Alcohol intake may be measured in grams or milliliters of ethanol, or in units of alcohol (e.g., each unit of alcohol in the UK contains approximately 8 g [10 mL] of ethanol). There is no standard European guideline, but the United Kingdom Department of Health recommends that adult men should not consume more than 3 to 4 units of alcohol per day and women should not consume more than 2 to 3 units daily. In the United States, however, a standard drink delivers about 12 to 14 g of alcohol, and the U.S. Department of Agriculture recommends that men should not drink more than 1 to 2 drinks per day and that women should not exceed 1 drink per day. These recommendations provide a guide to the everyday use of alcohol, but the problems associated with alcohol more often arise from "binge" drinking on specific occasions, and in football this can typically occurs during the postmatch period. This type of drinking is a potential risk for the players' postmatch recovery, as well as more generally for their well-being, health, and reputation if the drinking becomes habitual.

The actions of alcohol on the central nervous system result in decrements in skill and in behavioral changes that may have adverse effects on performance. There is also evidence of dose-dependent decrements in endurance capacity. Although the mechanisms are not well understood, the aftermath of alcohol use (hangover) may also adversely affect performance for many hours after intoxication. It appears unlikely that the intake of 1 to 2 standard drinks will have negative effects in most habitual drinkers, but all players should certainly avoid a heavy intake of alcohol on the night before a match.

The most important problem associated with the excessive consumption of alcohol after exercise is that it may result in various risky behaviors. Alcohol intoxication may make the player forget about following sound recovery practices such as appropriate treatment for injuries, adequate sleep, or optimal eating and drinking. Alcohol may displace carbohydrate from the diet at a time when restoration of glycogen stores should be a priority. It can also impair protein synthesis and thus compromise the adaptations that should follow a training session. The need for other important nutrients may be neglected while the player is consuming large amounts of alcohol, or sleeping off the hangover next day. An intoxicated athlete also often succumbs to high-risk activities, leading to accidents, violence, or other antisocial behavior. Negative outcomes can range from the tarnishing of a reputation to serious (and sometimes fatal) injury.

Before consuming any alcohol after a match, the player should consume a meal or snack to replace carbohydrate, fluid, and protein. This snack or meal will start the recovery process. Food intake will also help to reduce the rate of alcohol absorption and thus reduce the rate of intoxication. Once postexercise recovery priorities have been addressed, the player who chooses to drink should only be encouraged to do so "in moderation" and doctors should always try to be aware of, and prevent players from, overuse of alcohol. Drink-driving education messages in various countries may provide a guide to

what is considered sensible, and to well-paced drinking in general.

### 4.3.6 Vitamins, Minerals, and Micronutrients

A varied diet that meets energy needs and is based largely on nutrient-rich choices such as vegetables, fruits, beans, legumes, cereals, lean meats, fish, and dairy foods should ensure an adequate intake of vitamins and minerals. Excluding any of these food groups means that more careful food choices must be made. For several hours after heavy exertion, components of both the innate and adaptive immune system exhibit suppressed function, but a varied diet eaten in adequate amounts will provide all the nutrients needed to maintain a healthy immune system. Adequate intakes of energy and carbohydrate supplementation are also essential during periods of particularly hard training to sustain immune function.

### 4.3.7 Supplements

The use of dietary supplements is widespread in football at all levels, but the indiscriminate use of dietary supplements is strongly discouraged. A few supplements may bring some benefits to some players in specific situations, but supplements also carry risks to health and performance as well as the possibility of an Anti-Doping Rule Violations (ADRV). Supplements should be used only on the advice of a qualified sports nutrition professional. This topic is covered in more detail in Chapter 6.

### 4.3.8 The Pregame Meal

Most players appreciate the need to rest and eat well during the days prior to an important match, but questions arise regarding how much to eat, what type of food, and when is the best time for the pregame meal. Carbohydrate is the key energy-providing nutrient that must be optimized during the days leading up to and including the day of competition. Players who start a game with low glycogen stores are likely to end up being substituted before the end of the game. Attention should also be given to optimizing water and salt levels in the body. However, during the 2 to 4 days prior to a competition, a player's need for protein and fat, as well as most other nutrients, typically does not increase above the levels that are recommended for normal moderate-level training. Nutrition on match day is all about performance and this is often where tailor-made sports foods can help to meet special match needs more practically than everyday foods. Experienced players will know what works best for them, and they should be encouraged to follow their preferences, provided there is no evidence that their preferences are in any way harmful.

Players who train and compete intensely may benefit from reduced training loads and "carbohydrate loading" for a few days before a big game. This practice is common in endurance sports where competition is infrequent, but is less so in football. Very high glycogen levels may not be beneficial, but players starting a game with an inadequate glycogen store are unlikely to perform at their best, so it seems wise to ensure that glycogen levels are at least moderate to high. Eating a large amount of carbohydrate (about 8–10 g/kg of body weight per day; see below) at the same time that training intensity and duration are reduced will lead to very high levels of muscle glycogen stores within 2 to 3 days.

An example of 1 day of a carbohydrate loading diet providing 630 g of carbohydrate* (i.e., to provide 9 g/kg carbohydrate for a player weighing 70 kg) is provided in **Table 4.1**.

Players sometimes find a favorite precompetition meal that not only provides extra energy during the match, but also feels "right" in terms of curbing hunger, quieting their stomach, and being convenient and practical. For many players, a familiar prematch routine is important and the last meal is often a central part of that preparation. Players should be encouraged to find out what works for them and to stick with this—provided that what they are doing is not actually harmful to their performance. In low-key competition, or for some players who do less running in a game (e.g., goalkeepers), the prematch meal need not be predominantly carbohydrate based. However, in intense competitions, players are generally advised to focus on carbohydrate-rich foods to provide a total of 1 to 4 g/kg body weight of carbohydrate during the 6-hour period before exercise.

The main "mistake" players might make is to eat only a small amount of carbohydrate (less than 1 g/kg body weight) during the hour or two before the game and then fail to consume any carbohydrate during the game. The small prematch carbohydrate meal "primes" the body to rely more heavily on blood glucose, but it does not provide enough carbohydrate to sustain the player throughout the subsequent exercise.

Five different examples of foods that each provide 140-g carbohydrate in a precompetition meal[a] (2 g/kg for a 70-kg player) are as follows:

- 2.5 cups of breakfast cereal + milk + large banana.
- Large bread roll or three thick slices bread + thick spread honey.
- Two cups of boiled rice + two slices of bread.
- Four stack pancakes + half cup syrup.
- Sixty-gram sports bar + 500-mL liquid meal supplement or fruit smoothie.

Players should drink sufficient fluid with meals on the day before competition to ensure they are well hydrated on the morning of the match. Players will know that they are not well hydrated if they produce only very small volumes of dark-colored urine. There is no reason to refrain from drinking water or carbohydrate-containing fluids during the hours leading up to play. The aim, however, is not just to drink as much as possible in the prematch period. We now recognize there are some dangers associated with excessive drinking, and that it is difficult to provide exact guidelines for fluid intake that suit all players. All recommendations should be treated as a starting point and adjusted for body size and the factors that influence fluid needs such as environmental conditions.

In hot weather, players should try to avoid too much exposure to outdoor temperatures in the hours before the game. A fluid intake of approximately 500 mL should be drunk during the 60- to 90-minute period before the start of the game. This will allow sufficient time for urination of excess fluid before the game begins. In training or competitions that cause heavy sweating without sufficient opportunity for fluid intake, players often benefit by drinking 300 to 600 mL of fluid during the 15-minute period immediately before the start of the event. These volumes should be scaled down for female and youth players with a smaller body size.

### 4.3.9 Regulations and Guidelines Relating to Matches Played in Extreme Temperatures

The regulations and/or guidelines of some governing bodies such as Union of European Football

| Table 4.1 | | |
|---|---|---|
| **Example of 1 day of a carbohydrate loading diet providing 630 g of carbohydrate** | | |
| Early AM | 150 g | 2 cups cereal with milk + 250 mL fruit juice + 1 banana + 2 thick slices toast + thick spread of jam |
| Late AM | 50 g | 500 mL soft drink or 750 mL sports drink |
| Midday | 150 g | 1 large bread roll + 1 medium muffin + fruit smoothie |
| Snack | 50 g | 200 g flavored yoghurt + 250 mL fruit juice |
| Dinner | 200 g | 3 cups cooked pasta + 2 cups fruit salad + 2 scoops ice cream + 500 mL sports drink |
| Snack | 30 g | 50 g chocolate |

*Foods added to balance a meal, such as sauce on the pasta, can meet needs for energy and other nutrients.

[a] Note that other foods may be eaten at the meal.

**4**

Associations (UEFA) and Fédération Internationale de Football Association (FIFA) allow for specific measures to be implemented to protect the health of players when competing in extreme heat or cold. These can include provisions such as (for heat) crushed ice at pitchside, sun shades over team benches, cold water provided on both sides of the pitch, and cooling breaks during the match, which can be called at the discretion of the referee.

## 4.4 Special Needs When Playing Away/Traveling

Professional football players are well-seasoned travelers, spending much time traveling and living far away from home. These trips are often short, but may involve longer spells of travel for tournaments or preseason tours. Competition is usually organized in a national or regional league that requires weekly or biweekly travel to matches. Frequent travel over long distances can pose a number of challenges:

- Disruptions to the normal training routine and lifestyle while the player is traveling.
- Changes in climate and environment that change nutrition needs.
- Jet lag.
- Changes to food availability including absence of important and familiar foods.
- Reliance on hotels, restaurants, and takeaways instead of familiar home cooking.
- Exposure to new foods and eating cultures.
- Temptations of an "all you can eat" buffet-style dining hall or restaurant.
- Risk of gastrointestinal illnesses due to exposure to food and water with poor hygiene standards.
- Excitement and distraction of a new environment.

A strategy should be in place to ensure that players can eat well while traveling for away fixtures. It is important to investigate food patterns and availability at the destination before leaving home. This may help in planning useful food supplies to take on trips that can replace missing and important items. The club nutritionist or team doctor should contact the catering organizers at the destination to let them know of special needs for meal timing and menus. There should be an eating plan for travel that incorporates the best of the available food supplies (e.g., airline catering, restaurants en route) as well as self-supplied snacks, and all members of the traveling squad should be fully informed about the arrangements that have been made. The enforced rest while traveling will reduce energy needs, but can create more opportunities for high energy intake if the player succumbs to "boredom eating." Suitable snacks should be available to limit the damage done.

When moving to a new time zone, players and key support staff should adopt eating patterns that suit the destination as soon as the trip starts. This will help to adapt the body clock.

There will be unseen fluid losses in air-conditioned vehicles and pressurized plane cabins, so a drink plan that helps maintain hydration should be in place. It is also important to find out whether it is safe to drink the local water supply. If risky, players should stick to sealed bottles of water and other drinks, or hot drinks. Be wary of ice added to drinks —it is often made from tap water. In high-risk areas, bottled water should be used when brushing teeth and players should avoid swallowing water when washing the face or showering. In high-risk environments, a rigid policy of sticking to food produced in good hotels or well-known restaurants should be enforced and everyone in the squad should stick to food that has been well cooked, and avoid salads or unpeeled fruit that has been in contact with local water or soil (**Fig. 4.5**).

## 4.5 Special Environmental Challenges

Football is a global sport played in every country in the world. Those who play may face difficult challenges when the environment is unfavorable. Football developed as a winter sport in northern Europe where the weather is seldom extreme and where most major cities are at, or close to, sea level. At high altitudes or at extremes of heat and humidity, the nature of the game changes and players face different challenges. This can be a particular problem when players living and training in cool climates travel for games in hot climates without any time for acclimatization. These challenges can be magnified when players travel for international games and are under the care of a doctor who does not know their history.

High altitude results in a loss of appetite, but there are unlikely to be major implications for most

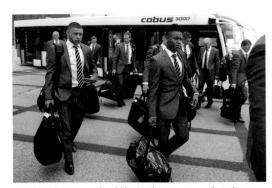

**Fig. 4.5** A strategy should be in place to ensure that players can eat well while traveling for away fixtures.

players at the moderate altitude (up to about 3,000 m) where most games are played. Hydration is important and players should be sure to drink plenty of fluids throughout the day. The drier air at altitude may increase fluid requirements and special care should be paid to monitoring hydration status. Because a move to a higher altitude may increase oxidative damage during exercise, athletes should ensure that their diet is rich in fruits and vegetables to provide essential antioxidants. For longer stays, such as tournaments, there will be an increased rate of red blood cell production, so the diet should contain plenty of iron-rich foods. It is worth checking iron status by way of a blood test before going to altitude.

When the temperature is high, we need to sweat more as we gain heat from the environment. High sweat rates over prolonged periods lead to large water losses and to some loss of salts. When the humidity is also high, the sweat cannot evaporate from the skin; it drips from the skin so no heat is lost, but we continue to sweat and so water and salts are lost at high rates. Those who normally live in cold climates will benefit from a period of heat acclimation before traveling to games in a hot climate, but this is seldom possible because of match schedules. Heat acclimation is achieved best by 60 to 100 minutes of modest exercise in a warm environment: about 10 to 12 sessions at intervals of not more than 2 to 3 days will achieve this, but any preparation is better than none. Players who are not used to hot weather must be aware of the need to make some changes to their routine:

— The warm-up should be shortened and carried out in the shade, with less clothing worn to prevent overheating and excess sweat loss before play begins.
— Extra fluids may be necessary, and cool fluids may be especially welcome, so insulated drinks bottles can help.

There is some evidence that lowering body temperature prior to running or cycling exercise may enhance performance in the heat, by either exposure to cold air, immersion in cold water, or ingestion of cold drinks, but it is less clear that players will benefit. Precooling will interfere with the normal prematch preparation, but the warm-up routine should be modified to prevent an excessive rise in body temperature before the game begins.

The effects of dehydration on performance seem to be greater in the heat than in cooler conditions, so it is especially important to be well hydrated before the start of training or match play. This means learning to look for signs of dehydration such as a gradual loss of weight, less frequent trips to the bathroom, and/or dark-colored urine. All of these are warning

signs of a need to drink more. Players should use meal times as opportunities to take more drinks. Those who know that they lose a lot of salt in their sweat might usefully add a little more salt to meals. Soups are usually a good source of both water and salt, and tomato juice has a very high salt content.

Players usually cope with cold weather simply by wearing more clothing in training and match play. Wearing gloves can greatly decrease heat loss from the hands. In cold weather, players tend to forget about their fluid needs thinking that their sweat needs are minimal, but sweat losses can still be substantial during hard training in extreme cold. Players wearing heavy kit may sweat as much in the cold as they do in the heat when they train wearing only shorts. The effects of dehydration are less serious in the cold than they are in the heat, so a higher level of dehydration is tolerable. This means that drinks may be focused more on providing extra carbohydrate. Hot drinks may be welcome at half time and after the game. Players may choose more concentrated carbohydrate drinks—sometimes up to 25% concentration—or even add carbohydrate gels and solid foods at half time. Experimentation in training will help the player to develop a match day routine that works for them as an individual.

## 4.6 Cultural and Regional Issues

Football is a truly international sport, and great players have emerged from every country in the world. Teams from different parts of the world will face different nutritional challenges, but none of these presents an insurmountable problem. A little attention paid to nutrition will pay big dividends in terms of better performance and better health.

Most teams will contain players from different ethnic, cultural, and socioeconomic backgrounds. On the field, they all play together and share the same aims and ambitions (and share the same physiology), but at home they are likely to have very different eating habits. Even though they all have broadly similar nutrition goals, an infinite variety of different food combinations can be chosen to meet their nutritional goals. All the essential nutrients can be obtained from normal foods, and variety is a key to meeting nutrient needs, but many different foods can be interchanged. Good sources of carbohydrate may be bread, rice, pasta, potato, couscous, or maize porridge. Protein will be provided by many different foods; the obvious foods are meat, fish, eggs, and dairy products, but bread, cereals, pasta, lentils, and beans are only a few of the other excellent sources of protein. The fruits and vegetables that are commonly available will differ from region to region, although many staples or favorites are exported around the globe. Our eating habits are much more international than they once were, and players can enjoy foods from different countries of the world.

The vegetarian player need not be at any disadvantage. These players, though, must be more aware of the food choices that they make. If there are no animal foods in the diet, then a vitamin B12 supplement may be necessary. Players who avoid red meat must pay special attention to ensuring that the diet contains enough iron from plant sources, and this should be combined with other foods that aid iron absorption: for example, iron-fortified breakfast cereals, consumed at a meal containing vitamin C (a glass of orange juice). Sufficient dairy products should be included in the diet to ensure an adequate calcium intake, but a wide range of calcium-fortified foods are also available for players with lactose intolerance.

There may be special circumstances that cause athletes to change their normal training and dietary habits. Muslim players normally avoid food and fluid intake during daylight hours throughout the holy month of Ramadan. This can mean that changes to training times are necessary to ensure that adequate hydration is maintained, especially in very hot weather and at high latitudes in summer. Where matches take place during Ramadan, players should be aware that prior preparation is necessary to ensure good liver and muscle glycogen stores and good hydration. Performance will not necessarily suffer if the player is well prepared, though this is easier to achieve when the whole team and support staff are fasting. When only one or two players are involved, special attention is necessary to ensure that the needs of these players are met.

## 4.7 Role of the Player, Support Staff, and Club

The player is the one who has to perform on the field of play, but all members of the support staff are responsible for ensuring that players can perform to their potential. Ensuring the right environment for training and in preparation for match play is a key element of that support and nutrition is a key element of every aspect of preparation. Players are responsible for what they eat and drink, and they are exposed to many sources of information that often provide conflicting advice. Most players and support staff have little nutrition knowledge and they generally have more pressing concerns, so nutrition is often neglected. A few will have their acquired beliefs that are incorrect, including an overemphasis on the importance of nutrition. Support staff must therefore provide guidance and direct them toward good choices. The club can help in this direction by providing suitable meals before and after training and games so that good choices become a habit. Players' use of dietary supplements, sports nutrition products, and sports drinks is also the responsibility of the club at professional level, and a clear policy should be in place to inform the players, and to protect the support staff.

## Suggested Readings

[1] Maughan RJ, ed. Nutrition and football. London: Routledge; 2007
[2] Maughan RJ, Watson P, Evans GH, Broad N, Shirreffs SM. Water balance and salt losses in competitive football. Int J Sport Nutr Exerc Metab. 2007; 17(6):583–594
[3] Maughan RJ, Shirreffs SM. Nutrition and hydration concerns of the female football player. Br J Sports Med. 2007; 41 Suppl 1:i60–i63

# Chapter 5

## Fatigue and Recovery in Football

*Grégory Dupont*

**5**

## 5.1 Introduction

In football, fatigue occurs in a variety of situations. This can be temporarily following short-term intense bouts of activity in both halves, toward the end of the match,[1] after the match, and during the season when the schedule is congested. A single match leads to an acute fatigue, characterized by a decline in maximal muscle strength,[2] which requires several days to fully recover. However, fatigue can also come from the repetition of matches particularly for successful teams. Some players can play up to 70 competitive matches per season. In these conditions, the number of weeks with two matches per week is greater than the number of weeks with one match per week. When the schedule is congested (i.e., two matches per week over several weeks), the repetition of matches can lead to a chronic fatigue among the players who play regularly, and incomplete recovery might result in underperformance and/or injury. Several studies have found that fixture congestion was associated with increased injury rates.[3,4,5]

Recovery strategies are therefore required to alleviate postmatch fatigue and to regain performance faster in order to reduce the risk of injury. However, before focusing on recovery strategies, it is necessary to analyze the factors leading to fatigue, to determine the fatigue mechanisms, the time course of recovery, and the level of scientific evidence of the fatigue markers currently used. This latter aspect will be addressed in the first part of this chapter. The second part of the chapter will deal with the recovery strategies that are available to reduce the magnitude of fatigue and to accelerate the time to fully recover.

## 5.2 Fatigue

### 5.2.1 What Is Fatigue in Football?

Football involves many physically demanding activities including sprinting, changes of direction and running speed, jumping and tackling, as well as technical actions such as dribbling, shooting, and passing. In performing these activities, a decline in performance, known as fatigue, can occur. Fatigue is a complex and multifaceted phenomenon, which depends on the type of stimulus, type of contraction, duration, frequency, intensity, and type of muscle.[6] It can be defined as any decline in muscle performance associated with muscle activity.[7] The activities performed by the players are not only physical. The playing environment is constantly changing, and players must collect and analyze information regarding the ball, teammates, and opponents before deciding on an appropriate response based upon current objectives (e.g., strategy, tactics) and action constraints (e.g., technical ability, physical capacity).[8]

Working on cognitively demanding tasks for a considerable time often leads to mental fatigue, which can also impact physical performance.[9]

In football, acute fatigue occurs during a match when a player has to repeat high-intensity actions, in the last quarter of the match, but it also occurs after the match and during the ensuing 3 to 4 days postmatch. Chronic fatigue occurs during congested schedules,[5] where the team may be required to undertake long-distance and repeated journeys for away matches.

Many factors can influence the magnitude of fatigue during and after a match:

— The fitness level of the player.
— The technical and tactical levels.
— The match status (i.e., whether the team is winning, losing, or drawing).
— The quality of the opponent (strong or weak).
— Match travel.
— The type of pitch (e.g., grassy, muddy, artificial).
— Some specific climatic condition, such as heat.[10]
— Atmospheric conditions, such as altitude.[11]

As a consequence, the amount of fatigue induced by football matches, with varying combinations of influencing factors, may vary greatly and affect the time course of recovery (**Fig. 5.1**).

### 5.2.2 What Are the Mechanisms Involved in Fatigue?

**Acute Fatigue**

*Fatigue during repeated high-intensity actions*: Football play requires the repetition of runs alternated with short to long periods of recovery. Goals or decisive actions are often preceded by accelerations, sprints, bursts of speed, jumps, and shots. However, when the recovery duration between these high-intensity actions is too short, the physical performance (e.g., the sprint speed) decreases. While the ability to maintain repeated sprint performance may be attributed to a multitude of factors, phosphoryl-

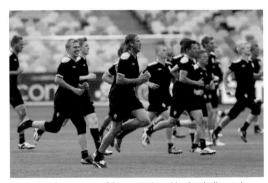

**Fig. 5.1** The amount of fatigue induced by football matches with varying combinations of influencing factors may vary greatly and affect the time course of recovery.

creatine availability and intracellular inorganic phosphate accumulation appear the most likely determinants. Moreover, the fact that both phosphorylcreatine resynthesis and intracellular inorganic phosphate removal are oxygen-dependent processes suggests that a high level of aerobic fitness may permit an enhanced ability to resist fatigue during this type of work. Following this type of repeated-sprint activity, peripheral, central, and supraspinal factors all contribute to the performance decrement and muscle fatigability of the quadriceps.[12]

*Fatigue in the last quarter of the match:* Fatigue occurring in the last quarter of a match is characterized by a decline in the amount of high-intensity running and may be induced by the depletion of glycogen stores.[10] Although this fatigue occurs toward the end of the match, it can also affect the postmatch fatigue, as muscle glycogen repletion after a high-level football match requires between 2 and 3 days when a specific nutrition plan is provided versus 4 to 5 days, when such a plan is not provided.

*Fatigue after the match:* After a football match, physical performance is significantly impaired: sprint performance over 20 m by 9%,[2] jump performance by 12%,[2] knee flexors maximal voluntary strength by 15%,[2,13] and knee extensor maximal voluntary strength by 25%.[14]

The recovery time course of physical tests (sprints, jump, knee flexors strength) after a match differs largely between studies, according to the population studied, with complete recovery requiring from few hours to more than 72 hours.[15] Unpredictable events that occur during a real match can explain this very high variability. In addition, running performance (total distance, high-intensity runs) is probably not the sole cause for postfootball match–induced fatigue.[16] Other variables, such as acceleration, deceleration, changes of direction, backward running, jumping, kicking, tackling, contact, and mental fatigue are probably more important in the postmatch fatigue mechanisms than the running activity profile. Nédélec et al[17] found that the number of short sprints (< 5 m) and changes in direction, requiring high acceleration and deceleration phases, were associated with significant neuromuscular fatigue that remain evident for up to 72 hours. Fatigue may be caused by factors within the muscle cells (peripheral fatigue) and diminished activation from the central nervous system (central fatigue). According to Rampinini et al[18], fatigue after a match is determined by a combination of central and peripheral factors both immediately after the match and within hours of recovery. Central fatigue seems to be the main cause of the decline in maximal voluntary contraction and sprinting ability, whereas

peripheral fatigue seems to be more related to increased muscle soreness and therefore may be linked with muscle damage and inflammation. Marshall et al[19] found that maximal voluntary torque decreased at the end of the half concomitant with reductions in central motor output to the biceps femoris, while no hamstring peripheral muscle fatigue was observed.

Although it is common to separate fatigue and muscle damage, the two phenomena overlap.[7] Muscle damage is likely to be a major consideration when attempting to explain the time needed to fully recover after a match. The repetition of changes of direction, accelerations, and decelerations throughout a football match may induce muscle damage. Muscle damage is characterized by muscle soreness, increased passive muscle stiffness, muscle swelling, morphological changes such as disruption and disorganization of sarcomeres, sarcolemma and transverse tubular system, and a prolonged reduction in maximal muscle force production.[20] A loss of muscle function lasting more than 2 days is a typical indicator of muscle damage, and muscle function measures are considered to be the best tool for quantifying muscle damage.[21]

### Chronic Fatigue

When the competitive fixture list is congested, there may be insufficient time in between matches for players to recover their psychological resources, potentially leading to lack of motivation and mental burnout. A congested schedule can be associated with frequent traveling, which may lead to the disruption of circadian rhythms (jet lag, sleep deprivation during overnight travel) and increase the level of stress induced by restricted motion, unfamiliar sleeping patterns, and poorer quality of sleep.

In summary, central fatigue seems to be the main cause of the decline in maximal voluntary contraction and sprinting ability, whereas peripheral fatigue seems to be more related to increased muscle soreness and therefore seems very likely linked to muscle damage and inflammation. Postmatch fatigue may be associated with glycogen depletion, muscle damage, and mental fatigue.

### 5.2.3 How to Monitor Fatigue

Management of fatigue during training and matches is essential in optimizing adaptation and performance. It should help reduce the risk of injury, illness, and overreaching. There are a range of different methods of fatigue management available to the fitness coach[22] including monitoring training load, physical tests, biochemical, hormonal, immunological assessments, questionnaires, and diaries. A balance has to be found between the number, the

5

frequency, and the order of the tests to make sure these do not affect the ensuing results. Familiarization with both the experimental condition and the battery of tests is another essential step to monitor fatigue. The balance between validity of the fatigue marker and its relevance to track the recovery process is also essential.

### Physical Tests

As fatigue is characterized by a decline in muscle performance, physical tests appear essential to measure the magnitude of the fatigue and the time required to fully recover. However, numerous hard and long physical tests performed at frequent intervals could induce a cumulative fatigue altering the recovery kinetics of the initial exercise. The physical tests could be short-sprinting performance, jumps such as the countermovement jump, and maximal voluntary strength. Although short-sprinting performance is an important determinant of match-winning actions, it could increase the risk of injury if assessed immediately after a match, as 70% of the hamstring injuries occurred during sprinting or high-speed running.[23] Jump tests appears safer, easy, and quick to implement. The reliability of these tests is high (**Fig. 5.2**).

Maximal voluntary strength testing also appears safer, but is not always easy to implement as these have traditionally been performed using isokinetic dynamometry, which lacks portability and which is time-consuming when testing a full team. However, some practical field-based tests can be considered with portable equipment such as force plate to test the isometric force[24] or specific equipment involving maximal eccentric contractions.[25,26]

### Physiological Markers

Heart rate variability at rest, following exercise, and during recovery has been proposed to monitor first the status of the autonomic nervous system, and then the positive or negative adaptations to training.

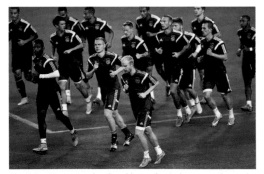

**Fig. 5.2** Numerous hard and long physical tests performed at frequent intervals could induce a cumulative fatigue altering the recovery kinetics of the initial exercise.

However, results from this method remain debated as many methodological constrains are required[27] and a consensus remains to be established.

### Biochemical Markers

Many biochemical markers are used to monitor fatigue. One of the most commonly used markers is the muscle proteins creatine kinase (CK) as it is easy to collect from a capillary sample and quick to analyze. However, the validity of CK as a marker of muscle damage is questionable[28] and reliability of the measure is low.[29]

Changes in hormones have also been studied following football matches. Cortisol is considered an important stress hormone and has an important role in both metabolism and immune function. Testosterone is a gonadal anabolic hormone that is required in muscle hypertrophy. However, the variability of these hormones limits their usefulness.[30] Immunological markers, such as saliva immunoglobulin A, present the same limitation: a low reliability.[31]

### Questionnaire

Questionnaires are simple to implement, relatively easy to analyze, and can be done at no cost. Monitoring training loads by Rating of Perceived Exertion (RPE) is a common method in football. It involves multiplying the perceived training intensity using a scale from 0 (rest) to 10 (maximal) by training duration in minutes.[32] The results represent the load, and it is also possible to calculate the monotony, which refers to the standard deviation of the training load during the week. The strain corresponds to the product of the weekly training load and monotony. This method is valid and reliable to estimate internal training load of football players.[33]

Some other specific questionnaires have been proposed in the literature, such as the Profile of Mood States (POMS) and the Brunel Mood Scale (BRUMS) to assess mood state, and also Recovery-Stress Questionnaire for athletes (RESTQ-Sport),[34] Daily Analysis of Life Demands for Athletes (DALDA),[35] and the Total Quality Recovery Scale (TQR),[36] to assess the level of stress and/or recovery. The limit of these questionnaires is that it requires the compliance and honesty of the players to avoid automatic response or the expected responses. Consequently, a moderate frequency of implementation with a small number of variable questions should be proposed to maximize the compliance.

In summary, markers used to monitor fatigue must be valid and reliable. Physiological and biochemical markers present some methodological limitations, are time-consuming, and expensive. Conversely, some physical tests such as jump and force, combined with some questionnaires, could be used to

**Table 5.1**

**An example of suggested fatigue variables to monitor in a team**

| Variables | Frequency |
| --- | --- |
| Rating Perceived Exertion (RPE) | Every session |
| Physical tests: CMJ/isometric force | Days after each match |
| Questionnaire of fatigue | Every week |
| Sleep | Every night |

Abbreviation: CMJ, countermovement jump.

monitor general changes in the fatigue and recovery status of players. An example of variables to test is proposed in **Table 5.1**.

Furthermore, as perceptual abilities (such as reaction time, decision-making, visual scanning, spatial awareness, and anticipation) are required to execute football-specific skills, psychomotor speed assessment could be an interesting addition, but requires further research to justify its usefulness.

## 5.3 Recovery

In order to reduce the gap between sport-science research and practice, a survey on the recovery strategies currently used in professional football teams has been performed.[16] Thirty-two professional clubs responded that the aspects they took into account for the recovery of their players concerned nutrition and hydration (97% of the clubs) and sleep (95% of the clubs), while the recovery strategies used after the matches or during the ensuing days were cold-water immersion and contrast water therapy (88% of the clubs), active recovery (81%), massage (78%), stretching (50%), compression garments (22%), and electrical stimulation (13%). Following this survey, the level of scientific evidence justifying these recovery strategies on the change in the measured physical performance was reviewed.[16] In this chapter, only nutrition and hydration, sleep, cold-water immersion, and compression garments are considered as effective strategies to accelerate the recovery process.

### 5.3.1 Nutrition and Hydration

Rehydration, carbohydrate, and protein consumption after a match are effective recovery techniques for replenishing water and substrate stores, and optimizing muscle-damage repair. This is explained in more detail in Chapter 4.

### 5.3.2 Sleep

In elite football, players are frequently exposed to various situations and conditions that can interfere with sleep (e.g., playing night matches, bright light in the stadium; performing activities demanding high levels of concentration close to bedtime; use of products containing caffeine or alcohol in the period preceding bedtime; daytime napping regularly throughout the week; variable wake-up times or bedtime), potentially leading to sleep deprivation. Sleep loss is associated with reductions in endurance performance, maximal strength, and cognitive performance.[37] Significant relationships between sleep duration and the immune system have also been found. Cohen et al[38] showed that subjects with less than 7 hours of sleep per night in the weeks preceding exposure to a rhinovirus are about three times more likely to develop a cold than those with 8 hours or more of sleep.

A poor night's sleep may be compensated by a short postlunch nap. Waterhouse et al[39] found that a nap, followed by a 30-minute recovery period, improved alertness and aspects of mental and physical performance following partial sleep loss. The ability to nap for short periods during the day may be a useful skill for players especially during a congested schedule. Another strategy to improve physical performance could be to extend sleep quantity over multiple weeks. According to Mah et al[40], extended sleep beyond one's habitual nightly sleep contributes to improved athletic performance, technical skills, reaction time, and daytime sleepiness in basketball players.

A high-glycemic-index meal, which is recommended for rapid restoration of muscle glycogen stores, significantly reduced sleep onset latency compared with a low-glycemic-index meal[41] and was most effective when consumed 4 hours before bedtime compared with the same high-glycemic-index meal given 1 hour before bedtime. Some other nutrients such as those containing tryptophan[42] or melatonin[42,43] are also recommended to decrease sleep onset latency and/or to improve sleep quantity and quality. Doses of tryptophan, as low as 1 g, can improve sleep latency and subjective sleep quality; this can be achieved by consuming approximately 300 g of turkey or approximately 200 g of pumpkin seeds,[44] while high concentrations of melatonin are contained in tart cherries. As light strongly influences sleep, sleep strategies that support the natural environmental light-dark cycle (i.e., red-light treatment before sleep, dawn simulation therapy prior to waking) and prevent cycle disruption (i.e., filtering short wavelengths before sleep) could be recommended for elite footballers.

### 5.3.3 Cold-Water Immersion

Several meta-analyses have confirmed the positive effects of cold-water immersion on recovery of performance.[45,46] Cold-water immersion postexercise has been shown to provide worthwhile benefits on anaerobic performances, i.e., maximal strength,[47] sprint ability,[47] and countermovement jump.[48] The following protocol could be recommended to optimize the effects of cold-water immersion on recovery of performance: whole-body immersion lasting 10 to 20 minutes at a temperature of 12 to 15°C[46,49] immediately after the match or following a high-training-load session.[50]

### 5.3.4 Compression Garments

The principle of compression garments is to increase the pressure on the ankle and to decrease pressure on the midthigh in order to improve the venous return and thus reduce venous stasis in the lower extremities. A meta-analysis on the effects of compression garments on recovery following exercise inducing muscle damage was led by Hill et al.[51] Data were extracted from 12 studies, where variables were measured at baseline and at 24, 48, or 72 hours postexercise. Results indicated that the use of compression garments had moderate effect on recovery of muscle strength, muscle power, CK, and in reducing the severity of delayed onset muscle soreness. As studies did not have a placebo condition (i.e., using a garment, but no compression), a placebo effect due to wearing the garments should not be excluded. The use of compression garments may provide an

easy-to-use recovery strategy in a team. They could be useful during air travel, especially during long flight, to reduce the risk of deep vein thrombosis.[52]

## 5.4 Conclusion

As described in **Fig. 5.3**, the recovery protocol includes six steps and should start immediately after the match.

The first step is hydration: the mass of the players should be measured and compared to the prematch body mass in order to propose the appropriate quantity of fluid to drink (150% of body mass lost). The fluid should contain a combination of water and a large amount of sodium (500–700 mg/L of water). The second step consists of drinking a tart cherry juice and chocolate milk in order to restore glycogen, to reduce oxidative stress and inflammation, to stimulate muscle repair, and to promote quality and quantity of sleep. The third step is the cold bath. The players should immerse themselves up to the neck at a temperature between 12 and 15°C for 10 to 20 minutes to accelerate the recovery process. The fourth step is to wear a compression garment that should be worn until bedtime. The fifth step is to eat a meal high in carbohydrate with a high glycemic index and protein within 1 hour after the match

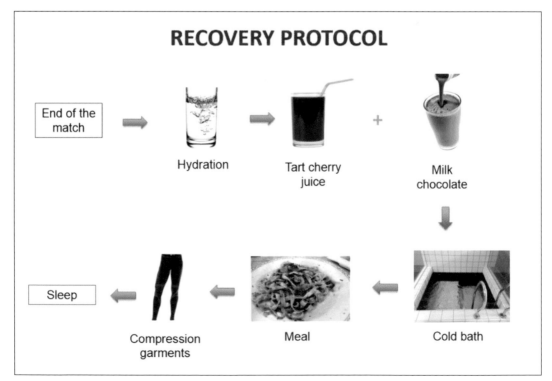

**Fig. 5.3**  Recommended recovery protocol.

(e.g., soup, well-cooked white pasta or mashed potatoes, chicken or fish, yogurts or cake). The last step is to have a good nights' sleep.

Although scientific evidence for the other strategies (active recovery, massage, stretching, and electrical stimulation) is still lacking in terms of their ability to accelerate the return to the initial level of performance, it does not mean that these strategies do not help to recover, but rather that the protocols implemented up until now have been unable to accelerate the recovery of physical performance. In addition, these recovery strategies are often isolated in the scientific papers, while practitioners revealed that recovery strategies are combined in recovery protocols. Finally, before prescribing recovery strategies, one must know the chronic effects of cellular to molecular adaptations.

## References

[1] Mohr M, Krustrup P, Bangsbo J. Fatigue in soccer: a brief review. J Sports Sci. 2005; 23 (6):593–599

[2] Magalhães J, Rebelo A, Oliveira E, Silva JR, Marques F, Ascensão A. Impact of Loughborough Intermittent Shuttle Test versus soccer match on physiological, biochemical and neuromuscular parameters. Eur J Appl Physiol. 2010; 108(1):39–48

[3] Bengtsson H, Ekstrand J, Hägglund M. Muscle injury rates in professional football increase with fixture congestion: an 11-year follow-up of the UEFA Champions League injury study. Br J Sports Med. 2013; 47(12):743–747

[4] Dupont G, Nedelec M, McCall A, McCormack D, Berthoin S, Wisløff U. Effect of 2 soccer matches in a week on physical performance and injury rate. Am J Sports Med. 2010; 38 (9):1752–1758

[5] Ekstrand J, Waldén M, Hägglund M. A congested football calendar and the wellbeing of players: correlation between match exposure of European footballers before the World Cup 2002 and their injuries and performances during that World Cup. Br J Sports Med. 2004; 38 (4):493–497

[6] Sahlin K. Metabolic factors in fatigue. Sports Med. 1992; 13(2):99–107

[7] Allen DG, Lamb GD, Westerblad H. Skeletal muscle fatigue: cellular mechanisms. Physiol Rev. 2008; 88(1):287–332

[8] Reilly T, Drust B, Clarke N. Muscle fatigue during football match-play. Sports Med. 2008; 38 (5):357–367

[9] Marcora SM, Staiano W, Manning V. Mental fatigue impairs physical performance in humans. J Appl Physiol (1985). 2009; 106 (3):857–864

[10] Mohr M, Mujika I, Santisteban J, et al. Examination of fatigue development in elite soccer in a hot environment: a multi-experimental approach. Scand J Med Sci Sports. 2010; 20 Suppl 3:125–132

[11] Aughey RJ, Hammond K, Varley MC, et al. Soccer activity profile of altitude versus sea-level natives during acclimatisation to 3600 m (ISA3600). Br J Sports Med. 2013; 47 Suppl 1: i107–i113

[12] Goodall S, Charlton K, Howatson G, Thomas K. Neuromuscular fatigability during repeated-sprint exercise in male athletes. Med Sci Sports Exerc. 2015; 47(3):528–536

[13] Ascensão A, Rebelo A, Oliveira E, Marques F, Pereira L, Magalhães J. Biochemical impact of a soccer match: analysis of oxidative stress and muscle damage markers throughout recovery. Clin Biochem. 2008; 41(10–11):841 851

[14] Robineau J, Jouaux T, Lacroix M, Babault N. Neuromuscular fatigue induced by a 90-minute soccer game modeling. J Strength Cond Res. 2012; 26(2):555–562

[15] Nédélec M, McCall A, Carling C, Legall F, Berthoin S, Dupont G. Recovery in soccer: part I—post-match fatigue and time course of recovery. Sports Med. 2012; 42(12):997–1015

[16] Nédélec M, McCall A, Carling C, Legall F, Berthoin S, Dupont G. Recovery in soccer: part ii—recovery strategies. Sports Med. 2013; 43 (1):9–22

[17] Nédélec M, McCall A, Carling C, Legall F, Berthoin S, Dupont G. The influence of soccer playing actions on the recovery kinetics after a soccer match. J Strength Cond Res. 2014; 28 (6):1517–1523

[18] Rampinini E, Bosio A, Ferraresi I, Petruolo A, Morelli A, Sassi A. Match-related fatigue in soccer players. Med Sci Sports Exerc. 2011; 43 (11):2161–2170

[19] Marshall PW, Lovell R, Jeppesen GK, Andersen K, Siegler JC. Hamstring muscle fatigue and central motor output during a simulated soccer match. PLoS One. 2014; 9(7):e102753

[20] Davies CT, White MJ. Muscle weakness following eccentric work in man. Pflugers Arch. 1981; 392(2):168–171

[21] Warren GL, Lowe DA, Armstrong RB. Measurement tools used in the study of eccentric contraction-induced injury. Sports Med. 1999; 27 (1):43–59

[22] Robson-Ansley PJ, Gleeson M, Ansley L. Fatigue management in the preparation of Olympic athletes. J Sports Sci. 2009; 27(13):1409–1420

[23] Ekstrand J, Healy JC, Waldén M, Lee JC, English B, Hägglund M. Hamstring muscle injuries in professional football: the correlation of MRI findings with return to play. Br J Sports Med. 2012; 46(2):112–117

[24] McCall, Nedelec M, Carling C, Legall F, Berthoin S, Dupont G. Reliability and Sensitivity of a simple isometric posterior lower limb muscle test in professional football players. Journal of Sports Science – Science & Medicine in Football J Sports Sci. 2015; 33(12):1298–304

[25] Opar DA, Piatkowski T, Williams MD, Shield AJ. A novel device using the Nordic hamstring exercise to assess eccentric knee flexor strength: a reliability and retrospective injury study. J Orthop Sports Phys Ther. 2013; 43 (9):636–640

[26] Sconce E, Jones P, Turner E, Comfort P, Graham-Smith P. The validity of the nordic hamstring lower for a field-based assessment of eccentric hamstring strength. J Sport Rehabil. 2015; 24(1):13–20

[27] Buchheit M. Monitoring training status with HR measures: do all roads lead to Rome? Front Physiol. 2014; 5:73

[28] Delextrat A, Baker J, Cohen DD, Clarke ND. Effect of a simulated soccer match on the functional hamstrings-to-quadriceps ratio in amateur female players. Scand J Med Sci Sports. 2013; 23(4):478–486

[29] Twist C, Highton J. Monitoring fatigue and recovery in rugby league players. Int J Sports Physiol Perform. 2013; 8(5):467–474

[30] Moreira A, Arsati F, de Oliveira Lima Arsati YB, da Silva DA, de Araújo VC. Salivary cortisol in top-level professional soccer players. Eur J Appl Physiol. 2009; 106(1):25–30

[31] Moreira A, Arsati F, Cury PR, et al. The impact of a 17-day training period for an international championship on mucosal immune parameters in top-level basketball players and staff members. Eur J Oral Sci. 2008; 116(5):431–437

[32] Foster C. Monitoring training in athletes with reference to overtraining syndrome. Med Sci Sports Exerc. 1998; 30(7):1164–1168

[33] Impellizzeri FM, Rampinini E, Coutts AJ, Sassi A, Marcora SM. Use of RPE-based training load in soccer. Med Sci Sports Exerc. 2004; 36 (6):1042–1047

[34] Kellmann M, Kallus KW. The Recovery-Stress-Questionnaire for athletes. Frankfurt: Swets and Zeitlinger; 2000

[35] Rushall BS. A tool for measuring stress tolerance in elite athletes. J Appl Sport Psych. 1990; 2:51–66

[36] Kenttä G, Hassmén P. Overtraining and recovery. A conceptual model. Sports Med. 1998; 26 (1):1–16

[37] Reilly T, Edwards B. Altered sleep-wake cycles and physical performance in athletes. Physiol Behav. 2007; 90(2–3):274–284

[38] Cohen S, Doyle WJ, Alper CM, Janicki-Deverts D, Turner RB. Sleep habits and susceptibility to the common cold. Arch Intern Med. 2009; 169 (1):62–67

[39] Waterhouse J, Atkinson G, Edwards B, Reilly T. The role of a short post-lunch nap in improving cognitive, motor, and sprint performance in participants with partial sleep deprivation. J Sports Sci. 2007; 25(14):1557–1566

[40] Mah CD, Mah KE, Kezirian EJ, Dement WC. The effects of sleep extension on the athletic performance of collegiate basketball players. Sleep. 2011; 34(7):943–950

[41] Afaghi A, O'Connor H, Chow CM. High-glycemic-index carbohydrate meals shorten sleep onset. Am J Clin Nutr. 2007; 85(2):426–430

[42] Halson SL. Nutrition, sleep and recovery. Eur J Sport Sci. 2008; 8(2):119–126

[43] Howatson G, Bell PG, Tallent J, Middleton B, McHugh MP, Ellis J. Effect of tart cherry juice (Prunus cerasus) on melatonin levels and enhanced sleep quality. Eur J Nutr. 2012; 51 (8):909–916

[44] Halson SL. Nutritional interventions to enhance sleep. Sports Science Exchange. 2013; 26(116):1–5

[45] Leeder J, Gissane C, van Someren K, Gregson W, Howatson G. Cold water immersion and recovery from strenuous exercise: a meta-analysis. Br J Sports Med. 2012; 46(4):233–240

[46] Poppendieck W, Faude O, Wegmann M, Meyer T. Cooling and performance recovery of trained athletes: a meta-analytical review. Int J Sports Physiol Perform. 2013; 8(3):227–242

[47] Ingram J, Dawson B, Goodman C, Wallman K, Beilby J. Effect of water immersion methods on post-exercise recovery from simulated team sport exercise. J Sci Med Sport. 2009; 12 (3):417–421

[48] King M, Duffield R. The effects of recovery interventions on consecutive days of intermittent sprint exercise. J Strength Cond Res. 2009; 23(6):1795–1802

[49] Halson SL. Does the time frame between exercise influence the effectiveness of hydrotherapy for recovery? Int J Sports Physiol Perform. 2011; 6(2):147–159

[50] Brophy-Williams N, Landers G, Wallman K. Effect of immediate and delayed cold water

immersion after a high intensity exercise session on subsequent run performance. J Sports Sci Med. 2011; 10(4):665–670

[51] Hill J, Howatson G, van Someren K, Leeder J, Pedlar C. Compression garments and recovery from exercise-induced muscle damage: a meta-analysis. Br J Sports Med. 2014; 48 (18):1340–1346

[52] Bartholomew JR, Schaffer JL, McCormick GF. Air travel and venous thromboembolism: minimizing the risk. Minn Med. 2011; 94 (6):43–49

5

# Chapter 6

## Nutritional Supplements

*Ronald J. Maughan*

## 6.1 Introduction

Many different factors contribute to successful performance in sport. Talent is undoubtedly the most important attribute of the elite player. It is easy to recognize but difficult to define, as the factors that combine to confer outstanding talent on an individual are varied and often not easily measured. Talent alone, however, will not produce a successful player and effective performance is achieved through a combination of complementary factors such as a sustained effective training program, psychological disposition, resistance to injury, and effective nutrition support. At a time when the world standard in the game is moving to ever-higher levels and the financial incentives are increasing accordingly, the player who wants to make it to the top and to stay there must explore all possible means of securing an advantage. At the highest level of the game, all players have great natural endowment and most are motivated to train hard in pursuit of success. As training programs become ever more demanding, bringing with them the risk of injury and stress, players will look to seize every possible advantage, and nutrition is one obvious area that can make a difference.

The foods that a player chooses can make the difference between success and failure. Good food choices will not make a champion out of the player who does not have the talent or motivation to succeed, but an inadequate diet can prevent the talented individual from making it to the top. A varied diet eaten in an amount sufficient to meet the player's energy needs should provide all the essential nutrients in adequate amounts, but not all players eat a varied diet and the total food intake may at times be restricted to achieve weight loss because of injury. This can lead to the potential for deficiencies of some nutrients: although severe deficiency is rare, a marginal deficiency (e.g., of iron) may be sufficient to compromise performance. Because the signs of an inadequate nutrient intake may be difficult to detect in their early stages, players are often tempted to take individual nutrients in a concentrated form to guard against the possibility of a deficiency developing. An enormous range of food components is also promoted as a way of enhancing performance, either directly through an effect on strength, speed, stamina, or mental focus, or indirectly through reductions in the risk of illness or injury.

To cater for the demand for specialist nutritional supplements for athletes, an enormous multinational industry has developed in recent years. This has been encouraged by a popular culture of supplement use among the general population in the belief that this can in some way compensate for poor food choices and the perceived stresses of modern life. One consequence is that use is often inappropriate: excessive, and potentially toxic, doses are sometimes used in the mistaken belief that more must be better. These beliefs are sometimes encouraged by support staff who lack training in nutrition but who believe that supplements can benefit players. Some clubs also receive sponsorship from supplements companies either as direct financial support or from provision of products, and it is expected that players will use these products.

## 6.2 Considerations for the Player

Any player contemplating the use of supplements should only do so after carrying out a careful cost–benefit analysis. On one side of the balance are the rewards, in terms of better health and performance, and on the other side lie the risks. The one-a-day multivitamin multimineral tablet is often seen as an insurance policy, "just in case" the diet does not meet requirements. These supplements are mostly benign, but this is not always the case. Routine iron supplementation, for example, can do more harm than good, and the risk of iron toxicity is very real. It has been estimated that, among the population of industrialized countries, twice as many men suffer from iron overload due to excessive use of iron supplements as from iron deficiency.

More exotic supplements, many of which have names that suggest an anabolic action and are marketed in a way that makes clear this intention, have become a prominent feature on the shelves of sports nutrition stores in the last decade or two. Some of these products make extravagant claims about building bigger, stronger, and faster muscles, repairing the damage caused by hard training, resisting infections and illnesses, and preventing chronic fatigue. Most are expensive, but for the athlete who is training to the limits, no price seems too high if the product performs as promised on the label. However, if we are to believe many top international athletes, they have paid a far higher price in recent years because of the presence in dietary supplements of doping agents that were not declared on the label.

Contaminated supplements are a very real risk and being labeled a drug cheat is something that no athlete wants, and something that no innocent athlete deserves. Although almost all involved in elite sport would agree that every effort must be made to ensure that any athlete who uses illegal drugs to enhance performance is caught and punished, most would also consider that the innocent athlete must also be protected. For reasons of legality, the existing World Anti-Doping Agency (WADA) anti-doping regulations, however, do not require proof of intent to cheat for an Anti-Doping Rule Violations (ADRV) to be imposed.

The offence lies in the presence of a prohibited substance in the urine or in an abnormal blood result: proving that there was no intent may be accepted as a mitigating factor, but it does not absolve the player from blame. Despite the need for this strict rule— namely, that doped athletes must be prevented from falsely using accidental contamination as an excuse to mitigate the length of a sanction—it is nevertheless unreasonable to expect players to be fully aware of all the nuances of the issues relating to doping control and of the risks of supplement contamination. For this reason, and due to the general complexity of the supplements market, doctors must put themselves in a position to be able to advise players appropriately and they can do this by ensuring that they are familiar with all of the issues involved.

In a team sport such as football where it may be decided by the medical team or nutritionist that supplements should be given to a whole team (either the same mix or a different combination per player), extreme caution must be taken by everyone involved. All team sports' regulations carry the WADA rule that if three or more players from the same team commit an ADRV in the same competition period, the entire team may be disqualified from competition (**Fig. 6.1**).

## 6.3 When Supplements May Be Useful

There is good evidence from both controlled laboratory and field studies and from the experiences of athletes that some supplements may provide performance and/or health benefits for some individuals in some situations. Where a player is identified as suffering from a deficiency of one of more essential nutrients, a dietary solution should be sought whenever possible. However, a prompt and effective solution may not always be possible, as players are often reluctant to change their diets. In severe iron

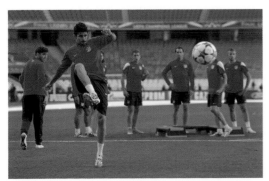

**Fig. 6.1** Where a player is identified as suffering from a deficiency of one of more essential nutrients, a dietary solution should be sought whenever possible.

deficiency, for example, use of a supplement is warranted and will, in most cases, bring relatively rapid resolution of the problem. Changes to diet can then be introduced more gradually to prevent a recurrence.

Where a supplement is used for this purpose, it should be sourced from a reputable supplier and should be used only at the therapeutic dose and for the shortest time consistent with restoring adequate nutrient status. Some athletes with restricted eating patterns, whether for religious, cultural, or ethical reasons, or because of a restricted energy intake during periods of weight reduction, may benefit from the use of a broad spectrum, low-dose multivitamin and mineral preparation, but again this should be obtained from a reputable source.

**NOTE:**

It is important to recognize that dietary deficiencies cannot be diagnosed on the basis of an estimate of the amount present in the diet. Every individual is different and most people need far less than the amount defined as the recommended daily intake: this is deemed sufficient for 98% of the population, so by definition, 98% of the population needs less than this amount. An assessment of nutrient status based on blood measurements or other biomarkers is essential for diagnosis of a deficiency state.

## 6.4 Supplements That May Be Effective

A small number of dietary supplements have been shown to be effective in improving performance in some specific exercise or sport contexts, but it must be remembered that few of these have been tested on football-specific tests. Where match play simulations have been used, the participants in studies have been recreational players or even nonfootballers. The evidence that footballers will benefit from these supplements is therefore very limited.

### 6.4.1 Creatine

Increasing dietary creatine can increase the creatine (and more specifically the creatine phosphate) content of the muscles: this provides a greater energy store for use during very high-intensity exercise and hydrolysis of the creatine phosphate can also help to neutralize the acidity that is produced in this type of exercise. The effects of creatine on performance have been extensively studied over the last two decades, and most, but not all, of the published studies show a beneficial effect on performance of repeated sprint exercise or of single bouts of high-intensity exercise lasting from a few seconds to a minute or two.

It has been argued that the balance of evidence does not favor a positive effect of creatine supplementation on anaerobic exercise performance, but that conclusion may be biased by studies where poor experimental design and lack of reproducible techniques have contributed to the absence of a measurable effect. It may also be biased by the inclusion of studies where the exercise test lasted more than 2 minutes. Benefits have most often been observed in high-intensity efforts of shorter duration and in multiple sprint tests where the recovery between sprints is short.

There may also be significant positive effects of creatine supplementation on gains in lean body mass and in muscle strength, which may be useful for some players. The experience of athletes seems to be that they perceive a performance improvement, and creatine use has remained popular. Not all players will gain the same benefit, however. There is some evidence that vegetarians may experience greater benefits: the vegetarian diet contains little creatine and these individuals start from a lower level of creatine in the muscles.

### 6.4.2 Caffeine

Caffeine can improve performance, though probably not as once thought through the stimulation of fatty acid mobilization and sparing of the body's limited carbohydrate stores, but rather via direct effects on muscle and on the brain. This would explain performance-enhancing effects in events of short duration where substrate availability should not be a limiting factor. There may be improvements in performance of tasks that require sustained concentration and there is some evidence that caffeine use may be effective in tasks involving skill and fine motor control. The effective dosage of caffeine is probably much smaller than previously thought and benefits have been reported with doses as small as 1 to 2 mg/kg, allowing athletes to gain benefits without some of the potential adverse effects of high caffeine doses. Possible risks include the diuretic action of caffeine and also difficulty in sleeping, which might be problematic if high doses were to be used for an evening game.

### 6.4.3 Bicarbonate

Bicarbonate, which is located primarily in the extracellular space, acts as a hydrogen ion buffer, helping to stabilize acid–base balance. In theory, this could be beneficial in high-intensity exercise where the production of large amounts of lactic acid causes levels of acidity in the muscle to increase to the point where they can contribute to fatigue: the increased pH gradient caused by the presence of high bicarbonate levels outside the muscle cells should facilitate the movement of hydrogen ions from the muscle cells where they are produced to the

extracellular space where the bicarbonate can neutralize them. High doses of bicarbonate taken before events where large amounts of lactic acid are produced can help improve performance: in practice, this generally means events lasting from about 1 to 10 minutes, though it might include longer events with frequent high-intensity efforts. Again, individuals should consider experimenting safely in training, and using only when a benefit is perceived.

### 6.4.4 β-Alanine

There are some promising recent results for supplementation with β-alanine. Supplement of the diet with β-alanine for a few days can increase the muscle content of carnosine, a dipeptide formed from β-alanine and histidine, which is an important intracellular buffer. Early results suggested that an increased muscle carnitine content can be effective in improving performance in events where acidosis may be limiting, though not all studies have given positive results. Various meta-analyses have come to different conclusions, in part because of different interpretations of the evidence but in part also because of the limited evidence available.

### 6.4.5 Nitrates

The potential effect of nitrate supplementation on health and performance has attracted much attention since the first reports in the scientific literature in 2007. A relatively small fraction of the energy turnover during exercise is used to do useful work, with the remainder appearing directly as heat. Thus, even a small increase in the efficiency of muscle contraction may be of major significance for exercise performance. Increasing the efficiency of muscle contraction would allow a greater work output for the same oxygen cost.

Laboratory studies show that ingestion of large doses of nitrate in the form of either pure sodium nitrate or beetroot juice (which, along with some other vegetables, has a high nitrate content) can result in a significant reduction in the oxygen cost of exercise and an improved performance. This would potentially benefit the football player by enhancing the amount of running that could be done in a game. Many athletes in various sports are now using various forms of nitrate supplementation, though there is still no complete understanding of the mechanisms of action.

## 6.5 World Anti-Doping Agency and the Prohibited List

The use of all of the compounds listed above is permitted by the current WADA regulations on doping in sports, even though the use of all dietary supplements is generally discouraged by international sporting bodies. The National Collegiate Athletic Association (NCAA), which governs collegiate sport in the United States, places a restriction on the use of caffeine in competitions that are held under their jurisdiction (but not in training): a urinary caffeine concentration in excess of 15 µg/mL is deemed a positive doping test.

Normal use of caffeinated products should not pose a risk that a player will exceed such a threshold, but the large individual variability in caffeine metabolism and excretion means that individuals who are subject to caffeine use restriction must be cautious when using high doses of caffeine. Players should also be aware that caffeine is present in many products, including tea, coffee, cola, and energy drinks as well as in many supplements that are promoted as giving increased "energy levels." In many cases, the presence of caffeine is not declared on the labels of these products. The use of combinations of these products may give an unexpectedly large dose of caffeine. Furthermore, caffeine is also consistently included on WADA's list of substances which are not prohibited but whose use is monitored by anti-doping laboratories.

## 6.6 Potential Health Risks

None of the supplements identified above has been shown to be associated with any significant health risk when used by healthy young individuals in the doses that have been shown to be effective.

**Creatine**: Concerns that have been expressed over the potential adverse effects of creatine use have not been substantiated by any evidence. There is no evidence of harmful effects on kidney function, nor is there an increased risk of muscle injury. Given that acute creatine supplementation in high doses can increase muscle strength and power within a few days, however, it seems sensible for athletes to be cautious in training when starting to take creatine. A sudden increase in weight lifted or in speed of sprints may well result in muscle strain or other injury.

**Caffeine**: Occasional use of caffeine in moderate doses is completely safe, though use in those who do not habitually consume caffeine may result in headache, nausea, and feelings of anxiety.

**Bicarbonate**: Apart from the possibility of acute gastrointestinal distress, which seems to be completely avoidable if the bicarbonate is taken in divided doses over the space of a few hours, there are no known risks associated with oral bicarbonate supplementation.

**β-Alanine**: β-alanine supplementation has been associated with paresthesia, a tickling or burning sensation on the skin, but this generally resolves rapidly and is not harmful.

**Nitrate**: Concerns have been raised as to the safety of high doses of dietary nitrate, but evidence for a range of beneficial effects on health is accumulating. However, the dose-response curve is entirely unknown, and overdosing may conceivably be health damaging, as with all nutrients consumed in excess.

## 6.7 Supplements and Contamination

Most athletes and coaches assume that supplements on sale in retail outlets are likely to be beneficial to health and performance and that the regulations governing their manufacture and sale ensure that they are safe for use. There is ample evidence, however, that the dietary supplements industry includes some companies that fail to observe the good manufacturing standards that should be applied. Third party contracting, whereby companies engage third parties to undertake manufacturing and packaging, means that there can be some lapses in quality assurance, even in the case of products from the most reputable of companies.

Various analyses of products purchased from retail outlets have shown that some products do not contain any measurable amount of the substances identified on the label, while others may contain excessive amounts. Because dietary supplements are not subject to routine screening by any regulatory authority, the extent of the problem is unknown. The absence of active ingredients seems more likely to occur when expensive ingredients are involved, presumably reflecting deliberate fraud. Fraud may extend to misleading information on product labels, with some claiming to be approved by the International Olympic Committee (IOC), Fédération Internationale de Football Association (FIFA), or other bodies. Such claims are totally false, but may mislead the naïve player.

The U.S. Food and Drug Administration (FDA) inspections of supplement manufacturing and storage premises routinely reveal a lack of good manufacturing practice, with some facilities failing to meet even the most basic standards of hygiene. This lack of quality control in the manufacture and distribution of supplements has caused the FDA to require manufacturers to close facilities and to recall products on a regular basis: an extensive database of these product recalls together with details of the reason for the recall can be found on the FDA website (see http://www.fda.gov/food/recallsoutbreaksemergencies).

Product recalls because of inadequate content include a folic acid product with only 34% of the stated dose. The FDA has also recalled products containing excessive doses of vitamins A, D, B6, and selenium because of potentially toxic levels of these components. Some products have been shown to contain potentially harmful impurities (lead, broken glass, animal feces, etc.) because of poor manufacturing practice.

In many cases, contamination probably results from poor quality assurance procedures, but there is also evidence of deliberate adulteration intended to transform otherwise ineffective products into extremely efficacious ones. In these cases, high doses, often exceeding the therapeutic dose, of potent pharmaceuticals have been found. While the resulting products are effective in achieving their stated aim, whether weight loss, muscle building, or other effects, they also carry significant health risks and the risk of an ADRV.

There has been a recent increase in the number of case reports of adverse health effects resulting from supplement use, and many of these have affected recreationally active individuals and amateur athletes. Hepatotoxicity seems to be the commonest problem. It was recently (2013) reported that dietary supplements now account for nearly 20% of all drug-related liver injuries presenting at hospitals, compared to 7% only a decade ago. Methylhexanamine (also known as 1,3-dimethylamylamine or DMAA and marketed as Geranamine) has been linked to a number of adverse events, including the deaths of two soldiers who suffered fatal heart attacks during a military training exercise in 2010 (*Army Times*, 2011), and its use has been regularly identified in positive sports doping cases in recent years. A female marathon runner who collapsed and died near the finish of the 2012 London Marathon had been consuming a commercially available product during the race and the coroner's investigation concluded that it had likely contributed to her death (*BBC News*, 2014).

It must be recognized that there are some major challenges in casually linking supplement use with any illness or fatality and therefore those cases that are confirmed are likely to represent only a small fraction of the cases that actually occur. In spite of the widespread reporting of these cases appearing in the popular media, there is no evidence of awareness of the risks among the general population or among athletes.

## 6.8 Supplements and Anti-Doping Rule Violations (ADRV)

The risk of a failed drugs test resulting from the use of dietary supplements has been recognized for more than a decade, and is a particular concern for athletes who are subject to testing programs for the use of prohibited substances. The presence in dietary supplements of agents that can cause an athlete to fail a test is well established, but limited data are available on the prevalence of contamination, as routine analysis for prohibited substances is not carried out by WADA or the supplements industry. The available evidence, however, is sufficient to indicate that the risk of the presence of a prohibited substance is very real and the risk has not been dramatically reduced since it was first recognized. Both independent analyses carried out by various laboratories and the analytical checks carried out by the FDA reveal a rather consistent pattern of contamination of supplements with pharmaceutical agents that are not listed on the label. The following products have recently been recalled by the FDA because of the presence of potentially harmful agents:

– More than 40 products marketed for weight loss.
– More than 70 products marketed for sexual enhancement.
– More than 80 products marketed for bodybuilding.

Weight loss products are most commonly found to be contaminated with anorectic agents such as sibutramine, causing powerful suppression of appetite after ingestion of an otherwise ineffective product. Sexual enhancement products are commonly found to contain analogues of Viagra. Bodybuilding products are most often found to contain anabolic steroids and related compounds. All of these undeclared additions are potentially harmful to health and most carry the possibility of a positive finding from a doping control test. Because their presence is not declared on the product label, the athlete has no way of knowing the risk. The principle of strict liability, however, means that ignorance of the presence of a prohibited substance in a product that is consumed is not an acceptable excuse and sanctions will still be applied.

Recent reports have indicated that the presence of even extremely small amounts of some prohibited substances can result in a positive test. Analysis of the urinary responses to the ingestion of small amounts of a nandrolone precursor (19-norandrostenedione) has revealed a high risk of a positive test: ingestion of a 1.0-µg dose of 19-norandrostenedione in 500 mL of water produced no values that were above the current WADA threshold for a positive doping test (2 ng/mL), but 5 subjects (out of 20) tested positive when 2.5 µg was ingested, and 15 subjects had urinary 19-NA concentrations exceeding the threshold when 5.0 µg of the steroid was ingested. These are extremely low levels of contamination.

## 6.9 Regulation and Risk Reduction Strategies

The problems with quality assurance in dietary supplements are not so much those of regulation but rather in the enforcement of the regulations that are in place. In almost every country, there is consumer protection legislation intended to ensure that products on sale are fit for purpose. In the case of supplements, this relates primarily to safety rather than to efficacy.

For most supplements in regular use, the available evidence is simply not sufficient for these products to be recommended, either to the general public or more specifically to athletes such as footballers. In many cases, this is simply because of an absence of any evidence at all: most supplements have simply not been subjected to rigorous tests to establish efficacy. There is also a need for critics of the use of supplements by athletes to be cautious: the absence of evidence of efficacy should not be interpreted as indicating an absence of efficacy. Most scientific tests can detect only relatively large effects: small effects that can be meaningful to the athlete are much harder to prove. Proving that a product has no effect, and therefore prohibiting its sale is much harder than simply not showing that it is effective.

Several programs are now in place that allow athletes who use supplements to make choices that will reduce the risk of a positive doping outcome as a result of using contaminated supplements. These programs cannot eliminate the risk entirely, but the sensible athlete will choose supplements that have been screened for the presence of doping agents by a reputable and independent company. The focus of these programs is on the testing of samples provided by manufacturers or distributors for the presence of WADA-prohibited substances. These sports-related programs are not complete quality assurance programs in that the presence of active ingredients is not usually verified. Athletes and those who are responsible for their care often see these programs as a guarantee of the integrity of products that have been tested, but it is important to recognize that a limited panel of substances is tested for and that the tests have limited sensitivity. In the Informed-Sport program in the United Kingdom, for example, the level of detection is set at 10 ng/g for steroids and 100 ng/g for stimulants, but some other schemes operate at different levels. For supplements that are consumed in large amounts, such as protein powders or drinks, a much more sensitive test is required than for supplements taken as small pills or capsules.

None of the current athlete-centered quality assurance programs for dietary supplements tests for the presence of the active ingredients. They are focused entirely on the presence of WADA-prohibited substances. Few screening programs test for contaminants other than stimulants and steroids, so the potential for problems resulting from the presence of other prohibited substances remains. Athletes should be aware of this and should not see these schemes as a guarantee that a product is safe to use. Rather, they should be part of a risk reduction strategy.

## 6.10  Foods and Doping Risks

Within the last few years, it has emerged that some foods may also pose a doping risk. The widespread use in some countries of Clenbuterol as a growth promoter in farm animals has resulted in the presence of residues in meat that can lead to an adverse doping outcome. This has been shown particularly in China and in Mexico. In the latter country, a large number of urine samples containing clenbuterol were recorded from players at the Under-17 FIFA World Cup in 2011. Other risks include the presence of the residues of veterinary steroids in meat products. This includes the presence of drugs administered to horses whose carcasses entered the human food chain. Awareness of the risks can help support staff minimize the possibility of an adverse analytical finding affecting one of their players, and risk reduction strategies such as avoiding certain types of locally produced meat when in known risk countries may be a useful strategy for the team doctor or nutritionist.

## 6.11  Other Risks

More recently still, a new risk has been identified for athletes. At least two cases are known where it appears that a pharmacist dispensing legitimate products to athletes has been responsible for a positive doping test because of the transfer of residues from a prohibited substance that has been prepared for a previous customer. Strict liability still applies even in this no-fault situation.

## Suggested Readings

[1] Consumerlab.com. 2014. Product review: weight loss supplement review. https://www.consumerlab.com/reviews/weight_loss_supplements_green_tea_7-keto-dhea/WeightLoss/

[2] Food and Drugs Administration. 2014. Beware of fraudulent "dietary supplements." http://www.fda.gov/ForConsumers/ConsumerUpdates/ucm246744.htm

[3] Hespel P, Maughan RJ, Greenhaff PL. Dietary supplements for football. In: Maughan RJ, ed. Nutrition and football. London: Routledge; 2007:141–163

[4] Informed Sport. 2013. Informed-Sport. What detection levels should supplements be tested at? http://www.informed-sport.com/faq#. Accessed November 27, 2013

[5] Maughan RJ. Contamination of dietary supplements and positive drug tests in sport. J Sports Sci. 2005; 23(9):883–889

[6] Maughan RJ, Depiesse F, Geyer H, International Association of Athletics Federations. The use of dietary supplements by athletes. J Sports Sci. 2007; 25 Suppl 1:S103–S113

[7] New York Times. (2013) Spike in harm to liver is tied to dietary aids. http://www.nytimes.com/2013/12/22/us/spike-in-harm-to-liver-is-tied-to-dietary-aids.html

6

# Chapter 7

## Anti-Doping

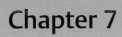

*Mike Earl and Zoran Bahtijarevic*

## 7.1 Introduction

Being the doctor of a modern football team is a demanding task that requires a devoted person, willing to subject themselves to mastering a wide range of skills, often outside those for which they are formally qualified. Pre-season examinations, periodical checkups, and constant fitness monitoring, together with diagnostic work and treatment of injuries and illnesses, make a team doctor one of the most significant actors in the machinery that supports a modern football team.

The wide scope of the role can be underestimated, and the work of a team doctor often only becomes visible when there is an injury or illness within the team. The expectation can be that the doctor should present a treatment solution in a matter of hours, particularly in the days leading up to a key match. This places pressure on the doctor to make informed decisions that comply both with their medical code of ethics to "do no harm" to a player, and with the code of ethics and rules of their sport (such as the anti-doping rules), while also trying to keep as many players as possible available for selection and performing to the best of their abilities.

The need for a doctor to understand the applicable anti-doping rules has become ever more important as players' monetary value and match availability value have increased. As the margins of victory and defeat are now increasingly narrow in elite football, and as teams look for any competitive advantage they can gain, the pressures placed on the doctor become ever more significant. Sometimes this may involve evaluating new measures to improve team performance, such as, for example, implementing new treatment programs for recovery and rehabilitation; however, extreme care must always be taken to ensure that medical work remains within the confines of the anti-doping rules. Ignorance and misunderstanding can quickly leave a doctor implicated in a doping case that can affect both theirs and a player's career. For this reason, it is essential that the modern football doctor has an understanding of anti-doping processes, and how to ensure that they and their players operate within the rules.

This chapter will set out the key points that a doctor should know with regard to anti-doping rules and procedures.

## 7.2 Rules and Regulations

The World Anti-Doping Code ("the Code") is the document that harmonizes anti-doping policies, rules, and regulations across international sport organizations and public authorities around the world. The Code works in conjunction with five International Standards, which are technical documents that cover key areas of anti-doping activity: testing and investigations; laboratories; therapeutic use exemptions (TUEs); the list of prohibited substances and methods; and the protection of privacy and personal information. For many years, sports federations, national anti-doping organizations (NADOs), and any other organizations conducting doping controls on athletes have been required to incorporate anti-doping rules which are compliant with the Code and International Standards into their statutes and regulations. The Code and International Standards are often updated and doctors should ensure that they are always aware of any changes when new versions are issued.[a]

For the football doctor, their responsibilities toward the Code and International Standards, and the overall anti-doping process may be summarized into the following key areas:

- Organization of the international anti-doping network;
- Types of Anti-Doping Rule Violation (ADRV);
- The List of Prohibited Substances and Methods (the "Prohibited List");
- Procedures for TUE approval;
- Doping control procedures;
- Anti-Doping Organizations' testing authority;
- Whereabouts rules.

Each of these key topics is described in this chapter.

## 7.3 Organization of the International Anti-Doping Network

The World Anti-Doping Agency (WADA) is the international body responsible for setting the anti-doping rules of sport and for coordinating anti-doping efforts across the world. Anti-doping organizations (ADOs), including international sports federations and NADOs, must comply with the Code and International Standards, and the awarding of, and participation in, major international sports events is generally conditional on compliance. All compliant ADOs (which include organizations such as Fédération Internationale de Football Association (FIFA) and Union of European Football Associations (UEFA) are required to implement anti-doping testing and education programs, and this is why footballers in any elite team will regularly have to undergo doping controls.

---

[a] Information related to the Code and International Standards provided in this chapter is correct at the time of publication.

## 7.4 Types of ADRV

The Code currently contains 10 types of ADRV, some of which can be only committed by players, and some of which can be committed by players and support staff, including doctors. It is important to note that even though football is a team sport, players remain individually responsible for any ADRVs committed under the Code.

### 7.4.1 Presence of a Prohibited Substance or Its Metabolites or Markers in an Athlete's Sample

This is the best known doping offence, where a prohibited substance or its markers are detected in a urine or blood sample provided by an athlete.

**NOTE:**
- This violation can only be committed by players.

### 7.4.2 Use or Attempted Use by an Athlete of a Prohibited Substance or a Prohibited Method

Here an athlete can commit an offence just by trying to dope. It is not necessary that the prohibited substance is detected in a sample, if it can be shown from other evidence that the athlete used or tried to use a prohibited substance or method to cheat.

**NOTE:**
- This violation can only be committed by players.

### 7.4.3 Evading, Refusing, or Failing to Submit to Sample Collection

This is a key offence for doctors to be aware of as it is they who often assist with ensuring players report to the doping control station (DCS) at the end of the match or during training sessions (or are at least made responsible to assist players once notified of selection). Any player who is deemed to have engaged in behavior such as (1) avoiding notification, (2) obstructing or preventing a doping control officer (DCO) or chaperone from notifying a player, (3) failing to report for doping control after notification, or (4) refusing to submit to a control when requested can commit this offence. It is therefore the responsibility of the doctor to try and discourage this type of behavior.

Often athletes who commit this offence because they are trying to hide doping will end up with a longer suspension for refusing to be tested than they would have received if they submitted to the test and tested positive (e.g., the use of substances included in the "specified substances" category on the Prohibited List can carry a lesser sanction than this offence).

**NOTE:**
- This violation can only be committed by players.

### 7.4.4 Whereabouts Failures

Out-of-competition testing has become a key part of international anti-doping operations in recent years and footballers are increasingly subject to whereabouts rules, sometimes with responsibilities to more than one ADO (e.g., UEFA and a NADO). Teams, and sometimes players individually, are required to provide regular whereabouts submissions to ADOs and some responsibility will often fall on the doctor or a member of the medical team to assist.

With the wide variety of whereabouts requirements that exist in football, for both teams and players, it is important to note that a whereabouts ADRV can only be committed by a player who is subject to some form of individual whereabouts requirements, whether that be individual whereabouts as described in the Code or partial individual whereabouts as required by some ADOs, such as UEFA.

A whereabouts ADRV is committed by a player who incurs three whereabouts failures in a 12-month period. A whereabouts failure can either be a failure by a player to make an accurate and complete whereabouts filing when required (a "filing failure"), or a failure to be available for testing during a daily 1-hour timeslot (a "missed test"). Whereabouts failures given to a player by different ADOs (e.g., a NADO and UEFA) can be combined, so players need to be particularly careful if they have to provide whereabouts information to more than one ADO.

As with all aspects of anti-doping, responsibility for complying with whereabouts requirements rests with the player. Even when a player's team provides whereabouts filings on the player's behalf, the player remains responsible for any mistakes, and it is the player who is suspended for committing a whereabouts ADRV.

Whereabouts considerations are described in more detail in Section 7.8 (p.81).

**NOTE:**
- This violation can only be committed by players. However, other individual player and team sanctions may exist under the rules of certain anti-doping organizations.

### 7.4.5 Tampering or Attempted Tampering with Any Part of Doping Control

The Code describes this offence as: "Conduct which subverts the doping control process but which would not otherwise be included in the definition of prohibited methods. Tampering shall include, without limitation, intentionally interfering or attempting to interfere with a doping control official, providing fraudulent information to an anti-doping organization or intimidating or attempting to intimidate a potential witness."

A team doctor could commit this offence, for example, if they were deemed to have obstructed a DCO in the course of their attempts to notify or test a player.

**NOTE:**
— This violation can be committed by a player or by their support staff (including doctors).

### 7.4.6 Possession of a Prohibited Substance or a Prohibited Method

Although players can be sanctioned for this offence, it is a particular risk for doctors in view of what may be contained in their treatment bag. As many substances on the Prohibited List are medications, a doctor must be careful not to carry prohibited items unless these are intended to be used in the course of legitimate treatment. However, the Code does provide some reassurance for doctors in the comment to Article 2.6.2 by stating that: "Acceptable justification would include, for example, a team doctor carrying prohibited substances for dealing with acute and emergency situations."

**NOTE:**
— This violation can be committed by a player or by their support staff (including doctors).

### 7.4.7 Trafficking or Attempted Trafficking in Any Prohibited Substance or Prohibited Method

Trafficking is considered by the Code to be selling, giving, transporting, sending, delivering, or distributing (or possessing for any such purpose) a prohibited substance or prohibited method (either physically or by any electronic or other means) by anyone subject to the jurisdiction of an ADO to any third party. This could be a doctor, a player, or other members of the team staff.

Again, to provide some reassurance for doctors, the Code indicates that the definition of trafficking "shall not include the actions of 'bona fide' medical personnel involving a prohibited substance used for genuine and legal therapeutic purposes or other acceptable justification, and shall not include actions involving prohibited substances which are not prohibited in out-of-competition testing unless the circumstances as a whole demonstrate such prohibited substances are not intended for genuine and legal therapeutic purposes or are intended to enhance sport performance."

Players dealing drugs or acting as intermediaries for a drug supplier would be subject to this rule, and all players should be made aware, particularly those who are young and impressionable. Social drugs such as cocaine, amphetamines, and cannabis are a significant risk, as are anabolic steroids, which are often distributed through gym and training environments outside the team setup.

**NOTE:**
— This violation can be committed by a player or by their support staff (including doctors).

### 7.4.8 Administration or Attempted Administration to Any Athlete In-Competition of Any Prohibited Substance or Prohibited Method, or Administration or Attempted Administration to Any Athlete Out-of-Competition of Any Prohibited Substance or Any Prohibited Method That Is Prohibited Out of Competition

This offence is another significant risk for doctors who will in the course of their daily work prescribe numerous treatments to players, some involving substances and methods on the prohibited list. TUEs are discussed later in this chapter, but their timely application and monitoring are essential to the modern football doctor in avoiding the commission of this offence. It is also essential that the doctor is familiar with the current version of the WADA Prohibited List in order that he/she is aware of when an exemption may be needed.

**NOTE:**
— This violation can be committed by a doctor and also by a player or by their support staff.

### 7.4.9 Complicity

The Code describes this offence as: "Assisting, encouraging, aiding, abetting, conspiring, covering up or any other type of intentional complicity involving an anti-doping rule violation, attempted anti-doping rule violation or violation of Article 10.12.1 (participation during ineligibility) by another person."

One risk inherent in this offence for doctors is the possibility that they could become aware of a player secretly using a prohibited substance. This can place the doctor in a difficult situation regarding disclosure, particularly when players are of such significant monetary value to their teams and the doctor is an employee of a professional team.

**NOTE:**
— This violation can be committed by a player or by their support staff (including doctors).

### 7.4.10 Prohibited Association

This is a new and complex offence under the 2015 Code, and players and doctors should be particularly aware of its implications with regard to players' personal entourages and external consultants who may be used/employed as part of the team's support network.

The rule is intended to prevent athletes associating with anyone who is currently suspended (or potentially going to be suspended) due to a doping violation and anyone convicted of a public offence that would otherwise constitute a doping violation if they were subject to anti-doping rules. The Code lists some examples of the types of prohibited association as the following: obtaining training, strategy, technique, nutrition, or medical advice; obtaining therapy, treatment, or prescriptions; providing any bodily products for analysis; or allowing the person to serve as an agent or representative.

The key point is to ensure that all staff working with the team (internal or external) are carefully vetted and that no one with a history of involvement in doping is allowed to work with players. Players should also be warned of the risks of committing this offence, particularly where there may be concerns about the individuals with whom they associate outside of their team environment. WADA publishes on its website a global list of athlete support personnel who are currently suspended from working with athletes, and teams should always check this before their organization employs new staff.

> **NOTE:**
> — This violation can be committed by a player or by their support staff (including doctors).

### 7.4.11 Consequences for Team Sports

The Code also contains collective sanctions that are specific to team sports. If more than two members of a team commit an ADRV during a competition period, an appropriate sanction is imposed on the team by the ADO or competition organizer. This may include loss of points, disqualification from the competition or event, or another sanction, and is imposed in addition to any individual sanction for the players who have committed the ADRV.

## 7.5 List of Prohibited Substances and Methods

The WADA Prohibited List is the document that identifies the substances and methods that are prohibited in all sports.

The list is generally published annually, and applies from 1st January each year (although new lists can be released at other times of the year). Doctors should be aware that the contents of the list change from year to year as new evidence is found on the effects of certain drugs, and as new methods of doping are identified. A review should therefore be undertaken at the end of each calendar year (or whenever a new list is released) to ensure that no players are using medication which is about to become newly prohibited.

### 7.5.1 Inclusion Criteria

Substances are included on the list when they meet any two of the following three criteria:
— Medical or other scientific evidence, pharmacological effect, or experience that the substance or method, alone or in combination with other substances or methods, has the potential to enhance or enhances sport performance.
— Medical or other scientific evidence, pharmacological effect, or experience that the use of the substance or method represents an actual or potential health risk to the athlete.
— WADA's determination that the use of the substance or method violates the spirit of sport.

Or as a general point:
— If WADA determines there is medical or other scientific evidence, pharmacological effect, or experience that the substance or method has the potential to mask the use of other prohibited substances or prohibited methods.

### 7.5.2 Defining In- and Out-of-Competition

The Prohibited List is split into substances and methods that are prohibited at all times and those prohibited only in-competition. In football, UEFA currently defines the in-competition period in its rules as starting 24 hours before a single match or the first match of a tournament, and finishing 24 hours after a single match or the end of a tournament, but this definition can vary for other competitions, depending on the rules of the competition organizer (e.g., FIFA or a national league). It is important for doctors to be aware that, as far as positive tests are concerned (i.e., an ADRV resulting from the presence of a prohibited substance or its metabolites or markers in an athlete's sample), the key is when a prohibited substance is detected, not when it is administered. Thus, a medication permitted for use, and legitimately prescribed and administered out-of-competition, which is then detected in a sample given by a player after a match (in-competition), could still result in the player incurring an ADRV.

As such, doctors need to be aware of the timing of treatment and average substance retention times for substances prohibited only in-competition.

In this context, addressing recreational social drug use by players can also be important, particularly for drugs like cocaine which are not prohibited (although clearly illegal) out-of-competition, but which could carry a sanction of between 2 and 4 years if detected in-competition.

### 7.5.3 Treatment Routes

The Prohibited List prohibits certain treatment routes, even if the substance itself is permitted, and doctors should always consult the Prohibited List carefully, particularly before giving intravenous infusions and/or injections, and before giving any anti-inflammatory injections such as glucocorticosteroids. Some ADOs and competition organizers operate "no-needle" policies and care should be taken to identify in advance when this may be applicable to an event in which a team is participating.

### 7.5.4 Checking Prohibited Status

WADA and many NADOs have their own websites where athletes and support staff can enter the brand name or constituent ingredients of a medicinal product and the site will confirm whether the substance is prohibited. Many such sites are now available as mobile phone apps which can greatly assist the doctor when quick treatment decisions need to be made, or when a TUE application needs to be completed.

The WADA app is available from most popular download sites, but NADO websites may sometimes be a more suitable source (where such sites are available) as the products listed are likely to be brand and country specific. The search will therefore be more accurate in terms of the products available in that country.

### 7.5.5 Traveling Abroad

International football involves significant worldwide travel, with clubs and national teams increasingly competing in countries outside of their own continent. Such travel poses another great challenge to a team doctor, certainly with regard to doping matters.

In principle, the doctor should try to avoid buying medications in foreign countries as these may contain prohibited substances which are not easily identifiable from the packaging (which may be in a foreign language), or which may not be contained in the same product when purchased in their own country. It is therefore always prudent for the doctor to carry small quantities of their own medications when traveling abroad (subject to any legal import controls on medication in the country being traveled to). In cases where medication must be obtained in a foreign country, the NADO of that country may be able to provide advice on prohibited status either directly or via its website, but available services may differ from country to country. The contact details of most NADOs are listed on WADA's website.

## 7.6 Procedures for Therapeutic Use Exemption (TUE) Approval

When a player has a health condition which requires medication, it is extremely important to check the prohibited status of the intended treatment. If the proposed substance or treatment method is prohibited, the player must obtain written approval from the relevant ADO via a TUE, and treatment must not start until this confirmation is received. Only in medical emergencies is a player allowed to start treatment before the TUE is granted, but there is no guarantee that in every case an approval will be granted retrospectively.

It is important to remember that although the doctor completes much of the TUE application form on the player's behalf, it remains the player's responsibility to ensure that they have a valid TUE for the use of any prohibited substance or method.

### 7.6.1 Preparing an Application

In principle, TUE applications should be made 30 days before a competition, but in sports such as football this is rarely feasible. Instead, as soon as the doctor has identified that treatment with a prohibited substance is needed, they should ensure that the TUE application form is signed by the player and submitted with as much supporting evidence as possible (e.g., imaging, test results, hospital specialist report), including details of all attempts to treat the condition with a non-prohibited medication. ADOs will normally return incomplete TUE applications to their sender, which inevitably delays the whole application process, so it is in both the player's and doctor's interest to submit a complete application file.

TUEs are approved for a specific period of time and for treatment only at the dosage specified on the approval, and doctors must be aware that any changes to a treatment regimen for which a player has a valid TUE will mean that a new application needs to be submitted before the dose changes; otherwise, the TUE becomes invalid. **Fig. 7.1** shows the TUE application process in its most basic form (without the appeals process).

Although it is always the player who is ultimately responsible for the application and timely renewal of a TUE, in practice this will usually be managed by

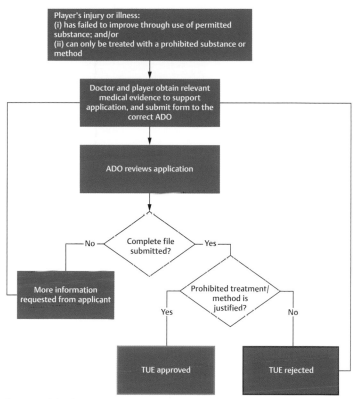

**Fig. 7.1** Simplified explanation of the therapeutic use exemption (TUE) application process.

the team doctor as they must complete the medical section of the application form. Doctors should always obtain any supporting medical documentation (e.g., consultation reports from a specialist, diagnostic tests, etc.) in a timely manner, which will prevent unnecessary delays to the approval process. The doctor should also strictly monitor the expiry dates of all TUEs held by their players and renew the application in good time if necessary. New applications must also be submitted in advance of whenever a change is made to a treatment regime for which a player has an existing TUE approval.

## 7.6.2 Submitting a TUE Application to the Correct Organization

TUE applications may need to be sent to different organizations at different times of the season. The correct recipient organization will depend on which competitions the player's team is participating in, and also whether the player has been included in a registered testing pool by an ADO. This is explained in **Table 7.1**.

Note that the above table applies to players registered to participate with European clubs and

| Table 7.1 |
| --- |

**Which anti-doping organization (ADO) should the player apply to?**

| Player/team status | New applications to: |
| --- | --- |
| Player registered for UEFA competition (team still competing) | UEFA |
| Player registered for FIFA competition (team still competing) | FIFA |
| Player registered for senior international friendly match | UEFA |
| All other times | NADO of the league in which the player's club competes |
| Player is identified as being part of FIFA's International Registered Testing Pool | FIFA |

*Abbreviations: FIFA, Fédération Internationale de Football Association; NADO, national anti-doping organization; UEFA, Union of European Football Associations.*

European national teams. For other players, care should be taken to consult the relevant regulations of the competitions in which the player is competing. It is also important to note that **Table 7.1** relates to new TUE applications. Should a player have an existing TUE approval from a recognized ADO, and they intend to compete in a competition under the jurisdiction of another organization, the TUE may need to be sent to the new organization for recognition prior to the player's entry into the competition. However, the exact application process will always be determined by the rules of the competition organizer/governing body and the doctor or team administrators should check this far in advance.

### 7.6.3  Review of Evidence

All TUE applications are reviewed by the TUE committee of the ADO to which the application is sent. The reviewing experts will be medical doctors, usually with experience of the sport. A TUE committee's role is to make sure that new approvals are only granted when the athlete can show that by a balance of probability **all** of the following WADA-defined criteria are met:

– The prohibited substance or prohibited method in question is needed to treat an acute or chronic medical condition, such that the athlete would experience a significant impairment to health if the prohibited substance or prohibited method were to be withheld.

– The therapeutic use of the prohibited substance or prohibited method is highly unlikely to produce any additional enhancement of performance beyond what might be anticipated by a return to the athlete's normal state of health following the treatment of the acute or chronic medical condition.

– There is no reasonable therapeutic alternative to the use of the prohibited substance or prohibited method.

– The necessity for the use of the prohibited substance or prohibited method is not a consequence, wholly or in part, of the prior use (without a TUE) of a substance or method which was prohibited at the time of such use.

Before submitting any application, doctors should consult the range of documents titled "Medical Information to Support the Decisions of TUECs" which are posted on WADA's website, and which provide the doctor with advice on applying for a range of common prohibited treatments.

It is important to note that rejected TUE applications can be appealed—to a national-level anti-doping appeals body, if the application was made to a NADO, or to WADA or CAS if the application was made to an international sports federations, such as UEFA or FIFA.

### 7.6.4  General Advice for Doctors on TUE Management

Doctors are advised to carry a copy (paper or electronic) of any valid TUE approvals with them at all times to be ready for a doping control, as players will be asked to document any recent medications and any valid TUEs which they currently hold. It is often sensible to make a few copies to be able to give one to a DCO in case of a doping control. The player should also get copies, which he/she should be advised to carry at all times (a scanned electronic copy on their mobile phone may be the best way to achieve this).

National team doctors often have a complicated task when preparing for an international competition, as many of their players will be playing for clubs in different countries, and as such the players will be under the jurisdiction of different NADOs. The best way to ensure up-to-date records for players is to establish good relationships with their club doctors, and to ask them to provide a copy of any TUE a player may have received while under their care. If this proves unsuccessful, one possible alternative approach is to directly contact the NADOs concerned and ask for copies; however, this may require compliance with national data protection laws.

Similarly, players may be given treatments while on international duty that the club doctor is unaware of, or at least uncertain of the medication used. The obligation here is on the national team doctor to ensure that they fully document all medications given, apply for TUEs when necessary, and keep proper records of TUEs granted to players under their care, and that they send this information on to the club doctor in good time. In addition, club doctors may benefit from reminding players before they depart for international duty to keep records of any treatment, or if not, to at least remember to try and photograph on their mobile phone any medications or treatments used on them by the national team doctor.

At all times, the doctor should remind their players to notify them of any new TUEs applied for by a different doctor or any changes to the status of an existing TUE.

More information about the TUE process should be available in the anti-doping regulations of the competition organizer or on WADA's website. Should competition-specific information not be available, the doctor should contact the competition organizer directly.

## 7.7  Anti-Doping Organizations' Testing Authority

Knowing which organizations have the authority to test your team can save time and a lot of unnecessary debate with a DCO. All DCOs should carry an identification card and documentation to verify their appointment by an ADO, and the team doctor should always ask to see this in the event of any uncertainty. Unless your team are formally (and in advance) advised that a different jurisdiction applies, the following ADOs have the right to test your players:

1. FIFA;
2. UEFA (while teams are in UEFA competition);

3. The NADO of a player's home country;
4. The NADO of the country in which a player's club is based;
5. The NADO of any country in which a team or individual player is residing (even temporarily);
6. WADA.[b]

Note that other organizations may also have the right to test players during a specific pre-event jurisdiction period (e.g., prior to a major event or competition).

Note that the fifth point should be considered in particular where players are sent abroad for treatment, or when teams travel on pre-season tours. Players need to be made aware that if notified of a doping control they must submit to the test. The identity of a DCO (in terms of the ADO they represent) should be verified by the team doctor if necessary.

## 7.8 Whereabouts Management

Out-of-competition testing is now commonplace in football, and providing whereabouts should be a routine activity for teams and players. However, it is important to note that different ADOs may impose different whereabouts responsibilities on teams and players. Individual whereabouts, as described in the Code, is intended for athletes in an ADO's Registered Testing Pool—those who compete at the very highest level in their sport, or who are considered to be the highest doping risk. Athletes subject to individual whereabouts have to provide, on a quarterly basis, details of all their training and competition schedules, as well as the address where they will be spending each night. They also have to provide, for every single day, an address and a 1-hour timeslot when they will be present at that address and available for doping control. Failure to provide either the required whereabouts information, or to be present at their stated address for the full 1-hour timeslot, is considered a whereabouts failure, which can, as described earlier in Section 7.4.4 (p.75), contribute to an athlete committing an ADRV. Depending on the risk priorities of an ADO, some players may be subject to these requirements.

It is more common in team sports for teams to submit collective whereabouts on behalf of their players and this is often referred to as "squad" or "team whereabouts." Here a team has to provide details of its training and match schedules, often on a weekly basis. Unlike individual whereabouts, a team whereabouts system is not described in the Code, and so

the information a team may have to provide will vary between ADOs, as will the sanctions for teams and players that break the ADO's team whereabouts rules. Usually, all players who are part of the squad are expected to be present at all training sessions unless the team notifies the ADO in advance of a player's absence. Some ADOs, such as UEFA for example, require players who are absent from any part of a team training session to provide, for the day of the absence, a 1-hour timeslot and an address where the player must be available for a doping control. Absent players who fail to provide the timeslot information, or who fail to be present where and when they should be, can incur a whereabouts violation. These violations are sometimes Code-compliant (i.e., they contribute toward a player committing an ADRV, as described in Section 7.4.4 (p.75)), sometimes not, depending on the regulations of the ADO. Team sanctions, such as financial penalties, may also apply under the rules of certain ADOs. Team whereabouts, either with or without the additional individual whereabouts requirements, are common at club level in many national leagues and in UEFA club competitions, and for national teams before and during major international tournaments (e.g., the FIFA World Cup or UEFA European Championship).

Good internal communication is essential to a team and its players effectively managing their whereabouts obligations. The following recommendations should be considered:

– That the persons(s) with overall responsibility for managing the submission of whereabouts are either with the main group of players at all times during training or are otherwise in regular communication with a team official who performs this role.
– That the team coach or manager immediately communicates any changes in training times or locations to the person(s) responsible for updating whereabouts.
– That all members of the coaching staff and medical team are briefed to immediately notify the person(s) responsible for updating whereabouts in the event that any players are scheduled to leave the training venue during the training times that have been notified to the ADO.

Sometimes individual players may be included in a Registered Testing Pool by an ADO different than that to which their team submits collective squad whereabouts (such as the NADO of their home country). In this case, it is essential that the player is supported by their team to ensure that changes to the team's training and competitive schedule are reflected in the player's individual whereabouts submissions (**Fig. 7.2**).

---

[b] For points 3,4 and 5, in some areas, a regional anti-doping organization (RADO) may conduct testing in place of a NADO.

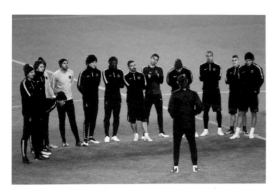

**Fig. 7.2** Good internal communication is essential to a team and its players for effectively managing their whereabouts obligations.

### 7.8.1 Minimizing Risk

Ensuring that coaches understand the concept of whereabouts, and are aware of the possible consequences of last-minute changes in training schedules without prior notification to the ADO, is crucial in avoiding whereabouts offences. If changes are not immediately communicated, DCOs may arrive to conduct testing without being informed of the change. At this point, it is too late, and the team and the player concerned may incur a violation.

It is also important to make players aware that they are ultimately responsible for updating their whereabouts, even though their team may do so on their behalf. It is also important to explain to players how personal whereabouts violations do not expire when they change clubs, and of their obligation to inform their new club of any existing violations on their record.

### 7.8.2 National Teams

When on international duty, players who are part of an ADO's Registered Testing Pool will usually remain subject to whereabouts rules, and it is therefore important that the national team doctor is aware of which players have continuing individual whereabouts obligations while under the national team's care. Furthermore, the national team may be required to submit collective or individual whereabouts for the team to an ADO such as UEFA or FIFA for the period in which the team are together, so it is also important that the communication structures referred to above are established within national teams.

## 7.9 Doping Control Procedures

Players and team medical staff should have at least a basic understanding of doping control procedures. This is primarily to ensure that all samples are collected correctly and with no risk of error or non-

compliance for the player, and also because both players and doctors have a professional obligation to support the work of ADOs in keeping football free of doping.

Doping control procedures are described in the WADA International Standard for Testing and Investigations (ISTI) and all ADOs should follow these procedures, especially the sample collection phase. Nevertheless, there are certain minor aspects of the procedures that are not prescribed in the ISTI, and so will vary between ADOs.

### 7.9.1 Compliance with Requests for Doping Control

A doping control is never convenient, whether it is at training where players have other post-training appointments, after a match, where the emotions of winning and losing can be tempered by a few hours' stay in a DCS, or at a place of residence such as a home or hotel where the intrusion into daily life can be unwelcome. However, for an ADO to conduct a truly effective anti-doping program, testing must be unpredictable and targeted at the time considered most likely to deter certain players or teams from doping, and to detect certain players or teams who may have been tempted to cheat.

The key aspect to consider with regards to being notified for doping control is that the DCO is not going to go away until the sample is collected. This means that the player either complies or refuses (the latter of which should be avoided at all costs). Considerable time can be saved for all involved if the player and the team staff accept the fact that, although doping control is never convenient, it is worth the inconvenience and effort to keep the sport clean, and that refusal or interference with the work of a DCO can result in as much as a 4-year suspension from football. The team doctor can play a key role in facilitating this process, and in setting the overall attitude of their team toward the doping control process. Doctors must avoid being seen to cause any obstruction or delay, particularly in view of the various Code offences that could be committed in serious cases.

### 7.9.2 Managing Players

Test distribution within team sport is becoming increasingly targeted, directed by science and intelligence factors, which are replacing the historical tendency to favor random testing. Consequently, players may need to get used to being tested repeatedly within what they may consider to be a short space of time, or to being tested more frequently than their team-mates. It can sometimes be difficult to reassure a player that they are not being treated unfairly, but the modern player can no longer assume that they will have a period without being tested once they have completed a test on a particular day. Players and teams can be chosen by ADOs for any number of reasons, and are still at times selected at random, but no ADO is under any obligation to disclose the reason for testing, or to justify how often they test.

### 7.9.3 The Key Stages of the Doping Control Process

#### DCO Arrival

DCOs should arrive without prior notice, and therefore it is essential that all team staff members are given a clear internal process to help facilitate testing. This should include ensuring that the doctor and other staff involved in the doping control are notified, and that the DCOs are given immediate and unobstructed access to the venue and players. This applies to both in-competition and out-of-competition testing.

For in-competition testing, the DCS should always be clean and available on match days even if the room is used for another purpose at other times. DCOs usually arrive before the start of the match, and so there is often a reasonable amount of time to prepare what the DCO needs. However, teams should never assume that just because no DCO has arrived by half-time that there will be no doping control. Reception staff at the stadium should always be prepared for one or more DCOs to arrive.

Upon arrival, DCOs must be given an up-to-date team sheet, and access to observe the players during the match either via a position in the tunnel or via a good standard seat that permits them quick and unimpeded access to pitch side (should a selected player be injured, sent-off, or substituted). Requirements for seat provision can vary according to the rules of the match organizer.

For out-of-competition testing at training sessions, doctors and team staff should be aware that the DCO usually has five main objectives on arrival:

— To identify which players are at the venue;
— To establish a suitable DCS;
— To complete a selection draw (unless all player selections have been done in advance by the ADO);
— To inform team staff of the selected players in order that they can assist with identification, and notification;
— To notify the selected players at the earliest possible (suitable) opportunity.

DCOs (or doping control chaperones, if used) must be allowed to observe the players in training when required. Players who have been selected for testing and who leave the training group early should expect to be tested immediately (**Fig. 7.3**).

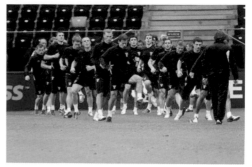

**Fig. 7.3** Players who have been selected for testing and who leave the training group early should expect to be tested immediately.

Doping controls may be conducted before or after a training session at the discretion of the ADO, and the timing depends usually, but not exclusively, on the type of sample to be collected. Blood samples collected as part of a biological passport program will usually be collected before a training session starts, as players are required to rest for 2 hours after exercise before they can give a sample, and this avoids unnecessary delays at the end of a training session. If controls are conducted after training, players are allowed to complete the session in which they are engaged, under observation by a DCO or chaperone, and notification will usually take place when the session finishes.

Out-of-competition tests can also take place away from training (such as at players' homes), and players must know what to do when a DCO approaches them. Most importantly, the DCO should never be delayed or obstructed once contact has been made with the player. Players' family members should also be made aware that a player could be tested at any time, and that they should never delay or obstruct a doping control.

#### The Selection Draw

If a selection draw takes place at a match or training session, this will be conducted by a DCO, usually witnessed by a member of team staff such as the doctor. Although procedures may vary by ADO, usually for in-competition testing, the draw will take place at half-time or during the second half, with the names of the selected players notified to the teams, for example, 15 minutes before the end of the match. In cases where players have been preselected by the ADO, the team representative will usually be notified by the DCO at a specified time during the second half. Doctors should note that targeted player selections are increasingly used by ADOs, and targets may be identified without explanation.

For out-of-competition testing at training sessions, the draw will usually take place immediately after the DCOs arrive at the training venue and before players finish training. When players are tested out-of-competition at a team hotel, the draw will take place as soon as possible after the DCOs' arrival.

## Notification

This phase involves the player being notified of their need to report for doping control by the DCO or a chaperone. Depending on the number of players being tested, the number of DCOs, and whether or not chaperones are present, the team doctor may be requested to help identify players for notification.

## Reporting

This phase starts after the player is notified of their need to report for doping control and ends when the player enters the DCS to provide their sample. Procedures may vary slightly by ADO; however, in principle, players must report immediately to the DCS on conclusion of the match or when notified at a training session, regardless of whether a chaperone is appointed (depending on the ADO). Usually, the player may not undertake any other activity, with the exception of flash media interviews within the tunnel area post-match. Under the rules of most ADOs such as UEFA, players cannot under any circumstances return to the team dressing room before reporting for a doping control. Non-compliance with this rule can result in a suspension, and in serious cases could lead to an ADRV, so it is essential that players are told that this rule applies and that they are reminded as often as possible.

## Declaration of Medication

Players must document on the doping control form any medication they have recently taken (the determination of what constitutes "recent" may vary per ADO, but usually means the previous 7 days). They may also be asked for the details of any valid TUEs they may have. Usually in football, this information is provided by the team doctor, but players must be briefed to consult with the doctor in the event that they are tested when the doctor is not there (e.g., if tested at home). Failure to accurately document medication does not necessarily lead to a doping violation, but accurate reporting can assist a player and the doctor if a positive test is returned for any prohibited substance.

## Sample Provision

This phase starts when the player selects their sample collection kit (a full kit for blood, and at this stage a sample collection beaker for urine) and provides their sample either in a toilet (urine) or at the table (blood) under direct observation of the DCO (**Fig. 7.4**).

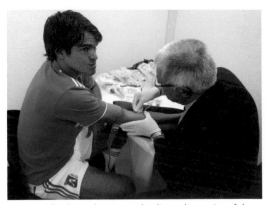

**Fig. 7.4**   Blood sample given under direct observation of the Doping Control Officer.

## Urine

Players must provide a urine sample of at least 90 mL. The DCO must observe the urine being passed, and so will ask the player to remove their clothing from the knee to the chest when providing their sample. If the player somehow tries to prevent the DCO from witnessing the provision of the sample (e.g., the player turns their back on the DCO), this could result in the player having to produce a further sample. If the player fails to reach 90 mL at the first attempt, the urine provided is stored securely as a "partial" sample and the process repeated when the player is ready again. Different ADOs may use slightly different procedures for partial sample storage, but the most important factors for the doctor and player are the security of the sample and a clear and secure labeling process.

Urine collection ends when the total urine provided reaches at least 90 mL.

## Blood

For blood testing, a needle is inserted into the player's non-dominant arm and up to five vacutainers (vials) may be attached and filled. The number and type of vacutainers used depends on the number and type of blood samples being collected and the type of analysis required, such as whether whole blood and/or serum is to be analyzed, or whether a blood passport sample is being collected. Up to three attempts at venipuncture will be made per player per doping control. If no blood is collected after three attempts, the player is excused from the blood test without further implications.

Doctors should be aware of players who have a fear of needles and should try to prepare accordingly, but this can never be used as a reason to excuse a player from a test.

## Dividing and Sealing Samples

For urine testing, the player chooses a sample collection kit and under the supervision of the DCO pours their urine sample from the beaker into an A and B bottle. At least 30 mL is poured into the B bottle and at least 60 mL into the A bottle. For blood testing, the vials collected are sealed in A and B containers, for serum and whole blood, or just an A container for a blood passport sample. All bottles and containers are securely sealed and placed in a box for transportation, with blood samples stored in a refrigerator or cooling box. It is essential that the player carefully checks that the bottle/container numbers recorded on their doping control form are the same as those on the bottles/containers and the box (**Fig. 7.5**).

It is important to note that the security of the sample rests in the bottle/container and not within the box or refrigeration equipment used to house the samples during transport. Once sealed, the sample cannot be tampered with, without the receiving laboratory being able to identify the tampering.

## Test for Specific Gravity (Urine Only)

The DCO measures the specific gravity (S/G) of the player's sample to ensure it is sufficiently concentrated to be accurately analyzed by the laboratory. This is done with the residual urine left in the player's sample collection beaker after bottles A and B have been sealed. If the reading reaches 1.005 or above (if measured with a refractometer; if a lab stick is used, it must be 1.010 or higher), this is fine, but if not, the player will be asked to provide another sample. The sample collection process will then be repeated until the player has produced a full 90 mL sample with suitable S/G.

One of the most common reasons for samples failing the S/G test is players overhydrating post-match. Unused substitutes are often at risk of this as they will drink too much while watching the match in the

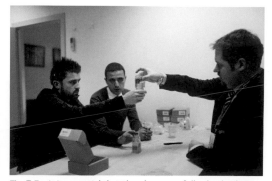

**Fig. 7.5** It is essential that the player carefully checks that the bottle/container numbers recorded on their doping control form are the same as those on the bottles/containers and the box.

hope that they can produce their sample quickly if they are selected. Some players also equate the amount of liquids consumed post-match with the speed in which they will start needing to urinate, which is obviously not correct, and again risks their sample being too dilute and failing the S/G test.

Players must also be aware that clear intentional attempts to overhydrate could be seen as a deliberate attempt to tamper with the doping control process. In extreme cases, this could even result in the player committing an ADRV.

## Completion of the Doping Control Form

Once all required samples have been provided, the player should complete and sign the doping control form, checking that all information is correct. If they have any concerns or comments about the doping control process, they should note them on the form at this stage. Players providing a blood sample for the biological passport will have to complete an additional form with a series of questions related to the passport.

Once this stage is completed the test concludes for the player, and they are released by the DCO. The player always receives a copy of their doping control form, which is nearly always given to the doctor, who should keep it in a safe place.

## Results Management

In principle, results should be communicated by the ADO that conducted the test directly to the athlete, but in football they are in practice usually sent to the player's club or national association. In most cases, ADOs will report results within approximately 1 month of the test (except for some tournaments where fast turnaround is essential), and the doctor should try to obtain confirmation that all results are negative. Be aware however that some ADOs only report positive tests and in some cases negative result confirmation will not be issued.

### 7.9.4 Points for the Doctor to Consider during the Doping Control Process

Although the majority of doping controls pass without incident in all sports across the world, on occasion, the sample collection process can have a significant bearing on the imposition of an ADRV. For this reason, doctors and players should be mindful of the following during the process:

- The DCS should be clean, private, and heated to a suitable temperature. Often this is the responsibility of the doctor's team (and ultimately the doctor), but it is essential to eliminate any risks of contamination of a player's sample, and to ensure that players are comfortable while they wait to provide a sample.

- No alcohol is allowed in the DCS under any circumstances.
- Players should always be given a choice of sample collection kit (e.g., beakers, lids, and collection bottles) and should never accept one that is handed to them by anyone else, including a DCO.
- Players, and their doctor, should always check that the sample collection kit they have selected is properly sealed. If there are any reasonable doubts, the player should choose another one.
- The DCO should not unnecessarily handle sample collection kit without the agreement of the player. This particularly relates to the dividing and sealing of samples.
- Partial samples must be stored securely with an appropriate labeling system to ensure that the sample is correctly attributed to the right player.
- Players and their doctor should always check that the sample numbers on the collection kit match the numbers recorded on the doping control form.
- Even on completion of the test, players should never leave the DCS without permission from the DCO.

Arguably the most important point during the doping control process for the doctor is filling in the test documentation, especially the box provided on the doping control form for comments. Regardless of how irrelevant an incident, irregularity, or complaint might seem, it should still be reported as it may turn out to be a crucial point in case of a disciplinary hearing if the sample is positive.

## 7.10 Other Special Considerations with Regards to Anti-Doping Procedures

### 7.10.1 Managing an ADRV

The worst outcome for any team is the possibility of being notified that one or more of their players has committed a suspected ADRV. Confidentiality from the point at which notification arrives is crucial (usually this is done by the ADO by telephone first, then followed up by letter), even for lower profile players, due to the interest in the sport from the public and media. As such, every team should carefully consider (1) who should be identified to relevant organizations (e.g., UEFA/FIFA) at the start of the season as the main contact for positive results and (2) who should be made aware of an ADRV within the team management structure.

The player should of course be notified as early as is possible, but great care should be taken to ensure that this is done in a sensitive and confidential manner. At major final tournaments (e.g., UEFA European Championship), a procedure must be put in place to manage situations where a player is provisionally suspended and is sent home from the tournament, particularly where the player is young and may require psychological support on their return. Usually a hearing will be held on-site by the competition organizer as soon as possible after the suspected ADRV is notified. Managing the national and international media can be a challenge in such cases, but a well-prepared media team can ensure that the best possible protection is provided to the player. The player's club should also be notified immediately via a trusted and prearranged contact (e.g., the team doctor).

The hearing and appeals processes are documented in competition regulations and are not discussed here, but the doctor should always be prepared to be required to testify at a hearing or an appeal, as ADRVs will in many cases involve the use of medication or supplements. This is another reason that a doctor should keep accurate TUE and treatment records to ensure that they are not unnecessarily implicated in a doping case for which they have no fault or involvement.

### 7.10.2 Anti-Doping and Minors

All doctors, and particularly those responsible for youth teams, should always bear in mind that they may be dealing with minors, as defined by national laws or by the rules of the competition in which they are competing. This means that the consent of a parent or a legal guardian should be obtained for every young player, covering not only medical conditions and the need for interventions when traveling without parents, but also the consent for a doping control and all its associated aspects (**Fig. 7.6**).

For most competitions, players under 18 years of age and their parents/guardians will be required to sign a competition-specific form in advance of the competition. The doctor should be aware of this in advance and should ensure that all forms are completed as a condition of the player's selection for the team. This is usually best obtained when the player

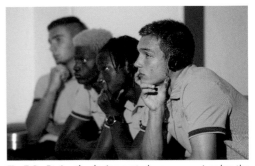

**Fig. 7.6** During the doping control process, a minor has the choice to be accompanied by a representative.

signs for the club, or before joining up with a national team. It is recommended to keep the signed forms with the players' identification documents that need to be carried with the team at all times.

Doctors should also be aware that during the doping control process a minor has the choice to be accompanied by a representative. The WADA ISTI 2017 notes that: "Athletes who are minors should be notified in the presence of an adult, and may choose to be accompanied by a representative throughout the entire sample collection session. The representative shall not witness the passing of a urine sample unless requested to do so by the minor. The objective is to ensure that the DCO is observing the sample provision correctly. Even if the minor declines a representative, the Sample Collection Authority, DCO or chaperone, as applicable, shall consider whether another third party ought to be present during notification of and/or collection of the sample from the athlete."

Doctors should discuss in advance with players whether they would choose to exercise this right or be satisfied to complete the process without a representative. Nevertheless, a good team doctor would ensure that either he/she or a reliable team representative (e.g., physical therapist or other member of the medical team) is present with their players in the DCS for the duration of testing. This will enable them to fulfill the role for all minors in the team as required.

Should a minor commit an ADRV, it is essential that proper support is provided to the player and their family throughout the disciplinary process.

### 7.10.3 Cooperation between Club Doctor and National Team Doctor

Although players spend proportionally much more time under the care of their club doctor than their national team doctor, continuity of care and support is essential. The primary role of this relationship will be one of ensuring that (1) players are fit to play for their national team and (2) return fit to play for their clubs; however, the need for good communication is essential for many aspects of anti-doping. As we have seen, medical treatment and TUEs must be documented and shared confidentially, but factors such as individual whereabouts and supplement consumption (where the national team and clubs have different regimes) are also important as neither the club nor the national association can afford to make mistakes that can lead to a player's suspension.

Sometimes cooperation may be difficult due to language, cultural, and organizational differences, but nevertheless the club doctor should try to obtain the contact details of national team doctors for all their players, and the national team doctor should seek to obtain the contacts of all of their players' club doctors. Only in this way can every change in medical status and every medication prescribed be communicated among the medical professionals in a way that respects the confidentiality and the rights of the player.

### 7.10.4 Managing a Player's Medical Network

It is important for the doctor to manage and be aware of (as far as possible) the network of sources from which players may obtain medical treatment and advice.

The doctor should keep notes of the following:
- All medications and supplements a player takes. The doctor should review with the team nutritionist or sports scientist whether all the supplements are necessary.
- Contact details of a player's family doctor or general practitioner, if any.
- Contact details of the player's dentist.

Team doctors should aim to contact all the player's external medical contacts (e.g., family doctor) at least once a year, either at the beginning of the season, or at the beginning of a new calendar year when new anti-doping regulations come to force. This can be a good opportunity to remind players of relevant anti-doping rules and provide them with the updated list of prohibited substances and any other useful information.

Players must also be regularly reminded to notify the team doctor of any treatments received outside of the team, and to discuss these with the doctor before use.

### 7.11 Summary

Given the wide scope of the role of the modern football doctor, anti-doping is often only considered as an occasional concern, and indeed most doctors and their players get through their careers without any doping-related problems. However, given the potential significance of a doping violation to the career of the doctor and their players, neglecting this aspect of the role can have significant consequences and as a result the points made in this chapter should always be carefully considered by any doctor working at the elite level.

Effective doctors are those who are organized, who understand the anti-doping rules, and who foster a professional attitude toward the process among all within their team structure, including the players. This can go a long way to ensuring that all involved can work together to achieve an effective anti-doping program for the sport, and a career without incident for players and doctors.

# Chapter 8

# Match and Tournament Preparation

*Ian Beasley*

## 8.1 Introduction

This chapter provides advice for the doctor on how to prepare best for away matches (particularly when traveling overseas) and finals tournaments. By the nature of football competition, most finals tournaments (e.g., the FIFA World Cup, UEFA Euro, Under-21 s, UEFA Women's Euro) will relate to national teams rather than clubs (with the exception of the FIFA World Club Cup); however, away matches in regional club competitions (e.g., Champions League, Europa League) also require considerable preparation on behalf of the team doctor.

## 8.2 The National Team Doctor (Medical Officer)

The national team medical officer (M.O.) performs an unusual role in terms of their management of players, as in effect they are required to support a player's optimum performance in the same way as a club doctor, but without the same day-to-day continuity in the management of a player's health and conditioning. As such, careful preparation for the period when players are under the national team doctor's care is paramount to ensuring the health and performance of the player to the optimum benefit of the national team, and to maintaining a good relationship with the player's club.

At clubs, access to players is taken for granted. There is daily contact with playing staff, and every aspect of every injury or illness is examined in great detail to ensure players are available for selection as soon as is safely possible.

The national team doctor has much less, if any, contact with players apart from when the players are with the national squad. In tournament-free years, this is approximately 50 d/y on average. This can rise to 80 to 90 days for the year if the team is at a finals tournament, and for some national squads may be even more if, for example, friendly matches and promotional tours are arranged.

Although there may not be regular doctor–player contact in the time between national team meet ups, the national team doctor should still be in communication with club staff on a regular basis, ensuring that the national team coaching staff are up to date with player status and availability for selection. It should always be remembered that the players are the employees of their respective clubs and that the national team "borrows" the players to represent their country. This necessitates careful planning and management by the doctor.

Elite players invariably carry a significant monetary value for their clubs; hence, some fear on the club's part is inevitable when allowing players to perform in an environment where they may suffer injury or illness, which could leave them unable to perform for their clubs. Hence, in the periods between international squad duty, it is imperative that the lines of communication with clubs are maintained by the national team doctor, allowing the club to feel confident in the national team staff. Wherever possible, the national team doctor should try to arrange club visits, with the aim of maintaining relations. This may be difficult for some doctors, especially where players may be at clubs abroad.

Preparation for matches (usually two games in a 10-day get-together) and tournaments (usually involving a much longer period together, perhaps in a different continent) requires different types of planning by the doctor, although both with a similar level of detail.

In each case, close attention should be paid to staffing levels to address the different challenges that the medical team will face and visits to venues must be carried out so that emergency action plans (EAPs) can be developed and reviewed by the whole multidisciplinary medical and science team (MDT). Regular meetings with coaching staff will allow support staff to plan any screening or monitoring that might be needed. This can then be organized around any training schedule.

## 8.3 General Issues

### 8.3.1 Planning Meetings

For all matches and tournaments, early planning meetings are essential. At the earliest opportunity, all parties involved in the management, logistics, and medical care associated with the national team should meet and broadly agree a project plan.

The following will apply to the medical part of the planning:
— Club contacts and visits.
— Roles and responsibilities of staff.
— EAPs for all venues/situations.
— Player health and immunization status.
— Precompetition medical examination/screening.
— Selection criteria.
— Acclimatization if appropriate.
— Planning of the pretournament camp.
— Facilities at all venues, e.g., pool, gym, area for ice baths, area for warm down, etc.
— Travel time to training and stadium.
— Arrival at venue.
— Debrief.

From this list, it should be possible to cover all issues, and to achieve the often difficult task of keeping everyone happy! At the very least if all involved know the issues that you will be dealing with, it can be assumed that they will be able to provide you with a better level of support.

### 8.3.2 Club Visits and Contacts for the National Team Doctor

It is not always easy to visit players' clubs, as in many cases, they will play in other countries from your own, and the cost of travel may be prohibitive. However, modern communication permits regular communication channels to be kept open, and can offer an easy and low-cost solution to help you meet your objectives of good relationships and good player management. Any updates on player status that you receive from a club can then be passed to the national team coaching staff/manager.

### 8.3.3 Roles and Responsibilities

As soon as is possible, the medical team should meet and agree their roles and responsibilities when with the team. You should be aware that extra staff can sometimes be needed for tournaments, so that the workload is shared with a larger group. In an ideal situation, these staff will be appointed early in the planning process, but this may not always be the case.

The agreed roles and responsibilities should include the following:

- Who is responsible for making sure each piece of equipment is carried when traveling with the medical team?
- Who will attend training and who will accompany players for indoor sessions if required?
- Which members of staff will assist with injury and extrication?
- Which staff members will assist with resuscitation if needed? Also, the automated external defibrillator (AED), the airway, cardiopulmonary resuscitation (CPR), and phoning the ambulance.
- Who will organize and run the mandatory resuscitation practice?
- Who will accompany players to hospital for investigation?
- Who will accompany anyone that needs repatriation?

Once these points have been agreed, the list should be circulated to all staff, including administration staff. It is important that any process should be understood by all involved so that decision-making and action are smooth whenever required. There must be flexibility, as there will be changes as time moves on. The most important thing is that change is appropriately and clearly communicated.

### 8.3.4 Emergency Action Plans

There should be an EAP in place for each venue at which the team is located during the period when players are with the national team. The EAP will ensure that all staff are aware of the processes to be followed should any medical emergency occur. The EAP should include the following:

- Knowledge of any current medical issues amongst the traveling party.
- Travel.
- Hotel(s).
- Training ground.
- Stadium.
- Local emergency service provision and how to contact the service providers.

### 8.3.5 Knowledge of Any Current Medical Issues in the Traveling Party

The national team, in any age group, attracts officials, press, security, and other staff to the traveling party. Whereas the playing staff are young, fit, and healthy individuals, the staff surrounding the team are often older, less fit, and may have ongoing health issues.

It is important that formal notification of current health status, with a list of medication taken, is submitted to the team doctor traveling with the team. Ideally, a decision on whether a person is fit to travel should be made with the team doctor, as the doctor can advise on medical risk while abroad, taking into account local conditions. The team doctor should make contact with all persons traveling, in order to assess the total risk, and whether any person may place an unreasonable burden on the medical team. If this is the case, it may be that a more detailed review of this person's medical condition needs to be undertaken. A letter confirming fitness should be supplied from their personal physician.

### 8.3.6 Travel

Travel administrative staff will have planned the travel arrangements. Contact should be made, and information on the mode and route of travel should be obtained by the team doctor. This should be done as soon as possible, once fixtures are confirmed.

Although it is often the case that travel plans change, it is usually timings that are most likely to be altered, often at the request of the coaching staff. The route and mode of travel usually remain constant.

You should have knowledge of the various hospital emergency departments that are situated near the route you might take, and you should ensure that you have the appropriate emergency medication with you, so that you may respond to any situation that might arise. This must include resuscitation equipment, including oxygen, and a defibrillator (AED) which should be with the team doctor at all times, as there is always the possibility that this equipment may be needed.

### 8.3.7 Hotels

Hotel choice is driven by the need to be near training facilities, and match stadiums. When administrative staff are making bookings, it should be routine that information regarding hospital locations are included in any briefing document that is circulated to medical staff.

Plans of the hotel should be supplied to medical staff by team administration staff, and routes of extrication should be identified with respect to the medical area, as well as other areas of the hotel that are occupied by the team and attached staff. Routes of extrication should be planned by the team doctor, and this may need to be done on arrival if a prior visit has not been possible. This should be done in conjunction with a generic risk assessment.

All this information should be disseminated to the wider medical team, and discussed at the first multidisciplinary meeting after arrival at the hotel (**Fig. 8.1**).

### 8.3.8 Training Venue

Once a training venue has been selected, the team doctor should (ideally) visit, and perform a risk assessment. This should include the following:

— Confirming the location of the nearest hospital and neurosurgical center.
— The siting of an ambulance if one is going to be present.
— The time it might take for an ambulance to reach the venue.
— Any issues surrounding extrication.

On arrival at the hotel, the team doctor should revisit the training ground to ensure there are no other issues arising. On arrival, the M.O. should check that the local emergency services are aware of training times, and confirm the presence of an ambulance at training, should this be the arrangement. At this time, confirm lines of communication.

All relevant information should be circulated to the wider medical team at the earliest possible opportunity after arrival at the destination.

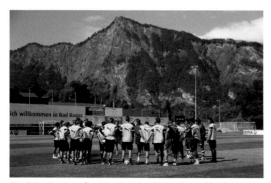

**Fig. 8.1**  Routes of extrication should be planned by the team doctor, and this may need to be done on arrival if a prior visit has not been possible.

### 8.3.9 Stadium

Once the stadium where the game is to be played has been confirmed, the team doctor should visit and perform a risk assessment. This should again include the following:

— Confirming the location of the nearest hospital and neurosurgical center.
— The siting of an ambulance if present.
— The time it might take for an ambulance to reach the venue.
— Any issues surrounding extrication.

In the case of a tournament or qualifying match, the team doctor should, in the first instance, liaise with Union of European Football Associations (UEFA) or Fédération Internationale de Football Association (FIFA) representatives on-site (e.g., the match delegate) to discuss the arrangements already in place. The team doctor should visit the medical and antidoping room at the stadium and confirm their location and that the stadium medical team are equipped as expected. This should ideally be done when the team train or visit the stadium on Match Day 1 (MD-1). The on-site ambulance should be inspected, so that the M.O. is aware of the facilities available, should they be needed. This will need to be done on MD-1, and on match day.

The team doctor should be in a position to obtain assurances that essential equipment will be available or be prepared to carry these items with them.

### 8.3.10 Local Emergency Service Provision

It should be straightforward to obtain the contact details of the emergency services from the host association representatives. For UEFA matches, it is a requirement that medical information is provided to the visiting team at least 2 weeks in advance. If this is not received, the host club/team should be contacted and if the information still cannot be obtained, the visiting team should contact UEFA.

Once received, the team doctor should contact their counterpart doctor in the host team if at all possible, and if language differences permit. This may be possible via the locally based team liaison officer. The host team doctor should inform the emergency services of the visiting team's accommodation, training venue, and arrival times.

If at all possible, a visit should be made to the local emergency unit or local private hospital to discuss admission, if necessary, for any member of the team or team staff. Privacy in accident and emergency, pathology services, pharmacy services, intensive care, and neurosurgical services are all important issues for the team doctor, as they will be the primary medical contact for all in the traveling group.

All the above information should be documented and provided to the wider medical team.

### 8.3.11 Player Health and Immunization Status

It is obvious that players' general health is a vital factor in performance. Players are as prone to illnesses as anyone else, and even high-profile players may have regular treatment for chronic diseases. The team doctor must make sure they have a supply of any regular medication taken by a player, just in case there is a lapse in memory or a baggage delay involving that players' luggage. Advanced liaison with clubs will make sure that any significant past medical history and allergies to drugs (and anything else) are recorded, and acted upon when and if necessary.

Knowledge of endemic diseases is also an important asset for the team doctor. If there is an immunization program that needs to be arranged with players' clubs, this should be planned at an early stage in advance of the match or tournament, so that adequate protection is afforded when there is potential risk. For example, if malaria prophylaxis is required, players in the squad may have experience of antimalarial drugs, and any accompanying side effects, so that the team doctor will be able to avoid using any particular drug that may cause these issues. This is a key part of the pre-event data collection process from players' clubs.

## 8.4 Co-Ordination of Precompetition Medical Examination/Screening

There are statutory precompetition player examination requirements for UEFA and FIFA tournaments, and some may exist for tournaments operated at national level. The type of screening is prescribed by the organization running the tournament, and usually includes cardiac screening.

If it is possible, part of the screening may be arranged at the players' club, which is another reason that a good club–country relationship is important. If this can be done, any issues identified during the examination can be addressed before the player has to report for international duty.

The national team doctor should be aware however that this practice may be unfamiliar to club team doctors not conversant with precompetition screening requirements for UEFA and FIFA competitions/tournaments. It is rare that any abnormality is found that might prevent the player's participation, as elite players are tested at clubs regularly. However, the prescreening remains an important tool in identifying an issue before something tragic happens to a player on the field of play. The team doctor must be aware that abnormalities may come to light that might prevent further participation in the planned tournament. He/she should ensure there are processes in place to deal with this very rare occurrence.

## 8.5 Selection Criteria

It may be asked "what has the medical team got to do with selection criteria?" and it is true that the medical team cannot comment on player ability or suitability for inclusion in a squad. However, the medical team can have an important role in advising on player status during the period leading up to selection.

Throughout the season, the amount of minutes each player has played is easily found on the internet or via other sources, and the doctor should aim to record the cumulative minutes played in an easily understandable format, for all to study. If the player uses Global Positioning System (GPS) at their club, similar figures can be collated for physical load. Such data give the manager/coach an idea of the possibility of fatigue in a player. This may not influence selection, but may help prepare the coaching staff for the fact that a player will not be able to train fully with the squad from the first day. This applies to players that are heavily involved in the latter stages of their national league or European competitions, which often means they have little or no break between the end of their club season and an international tournament. The aim of collecting this information is to inform rather than change the mind of the coach, but it does ensure that there will be fewer surprises upon meet up. This enables the medical and science staff to make sure the players who are fatigued get some rest, and that there are programs put in place for those that need more physical work.

In the build up to tournaments, there are preparation camps, which enable coaching and fitness staff to ensure that by the beginning of the tournament all players are at a similar level of fitness. The doctor should be prepared for situations where the coach wishes to select players who are still recovering from injury sustained near the end of the season, and most team doctors have been in a position where this has been the case. The role of the team doctor here is to give an honest and realistic opinion situation on any player. It should be acknowledged that there may not be enough staff to cope with rehabilitating a player at a preparation camp. It is possible that, if the player is deemed valuable enough, an extra member of staff, dedicated to this player's rehabilitation, may be recruited for this task only.

## 8.6 Acclimatization

Whether a friendly match or a major tournament, there may be differences in climate and/or altitude that are outside your players' normal experience. This then leads to a need for acclimatization, i.e., helping the players' physiology adapt so that performance is minimally affected.

There are many websites (e.g., http://www.wunderground.com) that will allow the team doctor to see what the weather was like at most venues for the last 3 years. This knowledge can help with temperature and humidity acclimatization. There are also many research articles on football at altitude; those published with the 2010 FIFA World Cup in South Africa in mind can be found in the *Scandinavian Journal of Medicine & Science in Sports* (Volume 18, Issue s1, August 2008).

The use of acclimatization chambers for both heat and/or altitude might be useful in any acclimatization strategy. However, there are time and economic factors to be considered in their use, and it has to fit in with the overall strategy of traveling to camps abroad, training programs, and the culture of the team. For example, some teams leave their departure for a match until the last possible moment, and adopt a "get in and get out" approach. In such cases, there is no physiological adaptation at the venue.

## 8.7  Planning a Preparation Camp

For one-off matches, this is rarely required. However, it might be the case that an important qualifying game is coming up, and the travel time is longer than normal. In this situation, the coach may wish to have a specified preparation camp, perhaps for 2 to 3 days.

More likely is that in the run up to a tournament, there will be the need for a period of preparation, both physically and psychologically (team building, etc.). This may incorporate some acclimatization, if this is a requirement for the upcoming tournament. A preparation camp is often planned by the coach based on past experience, or personal taste, rather than strict performance indices.

Ideally this camp should be planned with input from the multidisciplinary team and should include a medical component. Hence, once again, the possible venues should be researched, and ideally a summary prepared of the pros and cons related to each location. High-risk choices can then be discarded, and the coach can choose from the remainder, allowing him/her to retain some control over the decision without selecting a venue that may prove problematic for nonplaying reasons (**Fig. 8.2**).

A "recce" or advanced preparation visit to the site is very important, as no venue will exactly match the requirements of your team. Distance to training, gym equipment, meeting rooms, air conditioning in hotel rooms, food, and internet will all be

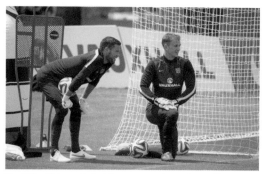

**Fig. 8.2**   Distance to training, gym equipment, meeting rooms, air conditioning in hotel rooms, food, and internet will all be considerations for the medical and sports science staff.

considerations for the medical and sports science staff. A decision will then be made as to whether the "wish list" that is made from the venue visit is possible from a budget and logistics point of view.

Once this part of the camp is over (or the tournament), it is important to review what worked and what did not. This will help you, or whoever comes after you, make the best decisions for future camps. Bear in mind that all this is aimed at maximizing the health and well-being of the players. It is easy for this to be buried in the large amount of activity involved in modern football.

### 8.7.1  Facilities at Venues

This follows on from the preparation camp, and it is important that the same process is carried out for all camps, so that the "flow" of work is duplicated, and players and coaching staff do not need to get used to new layouts. Of course, close duplication is impossible, but familiarity is important (without creating boredom!).

Incorporated in this is the travel time to stadium and training ground from the chosen accommodation (these will not always be the same). This is where one of the compromises lies. It is great to be near the training ground when in camp, but the hotel may not be as suitable as one a bit further away. Choose the hotel with the best facilities (as long as it is not too far!). Remember that training is usually for only 1 to 2 h/d with the rest of the time spent at the hotel, and boredom is a big factor. The players will enjoy the whole process better if they have a good hotel environment, which includes a functioning internet service as probably the biggest issue. It is possible to use "hot spot phones" or portable "hot spots" for internet access. Your team's information technology (IT) department should be consulted early on in this whole process to ensure that good internet connections are available not only for the players, but also for the medical and science teams, who rely on this for note keeping and analysis.

### 8.7.2 Arrival at Venue

On arrival, you will need to revisit your EAPs and ensure that nothing has changed since the planning visit. Any changes should be notified to all medical staff at these meetings, and to the rest of the team staff as applicable.

### 8.7.3 After the Get-Together

After each get-together, whether long or short, there should be a "debrief" meeting involving administration staff, medical staff, and sports science staff. This can be either face to face or via weblink. This meeting should review what was good and what did not work during the team's period together. Note that there is no "wrong or right" in this process, but there is always learning involved, and opportunities for improvement, which should be used as time goes on. The best way to record this is to have a list of venues, which includes EAPs, hotel facilities, food, rooms, etc., and training ground and stadia facilities, all stored centrally for use when required. Building such a resource will help with future planning as useful information gained should not be lost to the organization.

## 8.8 Medical Considerations

### 8.8.1 Medical Service Requirements

Many organizations/competition organizers have minimum requirements for medical provision in their regulations. Nevertheless, each club/association should develop their own medical standards based on their perceived medical requirements and availability in their own country. For obvious reasons, these should at least meet the minimum standards of the competitions in which your team will compete. There are some obvious "must-haves" such as an AED, but the team doctor should have all he or she needs to carry out his/her duties.

### 8.8.2 Staff Training

Resuscitation training is of utmost importance for all team medical staff. When you are with the national team, the staff working with you are unlikely to be the staff you work with every day of the week. It is imperative therefore that you practice resuscitation techniques and procedures for the removal of casualties from the pitch. At the beginning of the camp, make sure you allocate duties to your team (for instance, when at training, who will get the AED and oxygen?). If at a tournament, this practice should be done weekly, so that the whole team are aware of what they must do and feel confident to act as required.

A good knowledge of the current concussion guidelines (e.g., the Zurich consensus statement and UEFA and FIFA regulations) is important, and an education program should be delivered to the coaches and players so they understand the basic issues as below:

- If there is any suspicion of concussion, the player must leave the field of play. UEFA and FIFA regulations now allow the referee to give time for an initial on-pitch assessment.
- The decision of whether to take a player from the field of play is solely the doctor's.
- There is a gradual return-to-play program that will take *at least* 6 days

The idea of the education delivery is also to say "I will get it wrong sometimes." The coach and player(s) must understand that the doctor is fallible and could get the initial diagnosis wrong. It must be stressed that player safety is paramount and that the doctor must err on the side of caution.

### 8.8.3 Indemnity

Depending on your country of origin, the rules regarding indemnity insurance may vary. Medicine is a profession where things do not always go according to plan and if something goes wrong, and your employer or a player were to take legal action against you, it is imperative that you have appropriate insurance cover.

### 8.8.4 Drugs

All doctors will inevitably have a range of drugs that they would use, and these will vary depending on which drugs you like to use and are familiar with. If you are traveling, and your case of drugs is in the luggage hold/compartment of an airplane, for example, then it is important to have with you a small supply of anything you might need.

Some countries will have very strict rules on what they allow to be imported into their country and contacting the embassy of that country will help define exactly what the rules are. Exporting drugs via airports can be similarly troublesome, and you should make contact with your own emigration department or equivalent to make sure there are no difficulties at the airport.

### 8.8.5 Resuscitation and First Aid Equipment

When you visit a tournament or match venue, it may be possible to assess what level of equipment you will need to provide yourself (e.g., with UEFA MMR, it should be clear what equipment will be provided). However, for preparation camps, which can be at a hotel with an adjacent pitch, there may be no provision for such equipment, and it will be yours or your association's responsibility to ensure you have this with you. A similar situation applies for the other

8

equipment associated with first aid and pitch removal of players.

### 8.8.6 At the Stadium

For national qualification and tournament games, there is a statutory requirement to visit and/or train at the stadium on MD-1. This practice is usually followed for friendly games, but the situation varies. At UEFA matches, the official MD-1 training session is covered by the MMR, with services varying according to the level of competition (**Fig. 8.3**).

The doctor should ensure that an EAP is circulated to all team staff. This should be checked by the team doctor or someone nominated by them. For UEFA competitions, details of the stadium medical service and medical evacuation plan should be provided by the host team/association in advance of the match/competition.

For UEFA and FIFA matches, there will be a M.O. and pitchside rescue arrangements in place as standard. You should check on MD-1 that all equipment provided is of a standard that you would expect, and this check must be carried out before players enter for their warm-up. If there are any deficiencies, this should be mentioned to the match delegate, and remedied if possible. If not, alternative plans must be devised with your medical team, and all other team staff informed. If the match is not in a UEFA or FIFA competition, the host association, in conjunction with the stadium medical setup, will have their own emergency procedures, and you must confirm any differences in practice, and disseminate this information to the rest of the medical team.

On match day, it is important that you visit the referee's room and make sure that you agree on the rules regarding concussion, and any other issues that

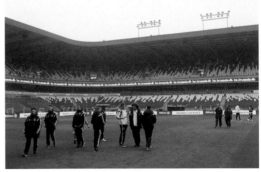

**Fig. 8.3** On match day, it is important that you visit the referee's room and make sure that you agree on the rules regarding concussion, and any other issues that concern player treatment and removal during the match.

concern player treatment and removal during the match. You should make sure that you introduce yourself to all stadium pitchside staff so that they know who they may be dealing with should an emergency occur. At this time, you must also check all the equipment they have and check again where the ambulance is sited. You should then check all equipment on the ambulance and pass any relevant information to your medical team.

### 8.8.7 Debrief

It is imperative that any lessons to be learnt *are* learnt. Performance on the field is out of the doctor's hands, but there are many things that impact on player availability and this is something the doctor can effect. No opportunity should be missed in evaluating the event, and in using this to prepare for the *next* event.

# Chapter 9

## Precompetition and Pretransfer Medical Screening

*Tim Meyer*

## 9.1 Introduction

The purpose of a general screening during eligibility examinations and pretransfer screening examinations differs widely. Whereas the focus during eligibility screening (usually once per year) is on the avoidance of fatal events and detrimental health effects due to regular high-level football play, pretransfer screening (scheduled according to when players change club) aims to assess the likelihood of a high participation rate in training and competition during the duration of the contract. Medical examinations should always have the health (short and long term) of the patient as highest priority, but reality in professional football may lead to certain additional obligations. The choice of examinations is mainly made on the basis of the above-mentioned purposes.

Prior to evaluating the benefits of various screening types, it is important for the doctor to be aware that precompetition screening is mandatory for all Union of European Football Associations (UEFA) and Fédération Internationale de Football Association (FIFA) competitions, and a list of specific tests must be conducted on each player as a precondition for eligibility. In UEFA competitions, requirements differ per tournament and per tournament phase (e.g., whether a team is qualified for a final tournament), and the doctor should check this carefully. Nevertheless, all elite players should be subject to an internal screening policy determined by their club or national association, which should be designed to protect the health of the player, and also their opponents and teammates (with regard to communicable diseases).

This chapter will review the different considerations in the screening of players for elite football, both for precompetition fitness/eligibility and for pretransfer signings. This will include explaining how the choice of examinations depends on the screening purpose. Although statistical considerations are relevant, screening decisions are not solely about sensitivity and specificity. Also, cost-effectiveness is an important issue that has to be valued against other aspects (like the potential public awareness of fatal events in very exposed players) and differs between countries.

## 9.2 Evaluating Statistical Issues Related to Examinations

Even allowing for the requirement to perform certain mandatory examinations as part of the precompetition screening, the doctor must also take several statistical issues into account to understand the background of the regulations. Likewise, this is necessary when deciding on which additional examinations to conduct. This should include considerations of sensitivity, specificity, and positive and negative predictive value.

- **Sensitivity**: The proportion of people known to have the disease, who test positive for it
  - = number of true positives/ (number of true positives + number of false negatives)
  - = number of true positives/total number of sick individuals in population
  - = probability of a positive test, given that the patient is ill.
- **Specificity**: The proportion of healthy patients known **not** to have the disease, who will test negative for it.
  - = number of true negatives/ (number of true negatives + number of false positives)
  - = number of true negatives/total number of healthy individuals in population
  - = probability of a negative test, given that the patient is healthy.
- **Positive predictive value**: The likelihood that a positive-tested individual really has the disease of interest.
- **Negative predictive value**: The likelihood that a negative-tested individual really does not have the disease of interest.

Screening tools should have a high sensitivity (to avoid missing diseases) which typically impairs specificity to a certain degree because there is always some trade-off between sensitivity and specificity. When sensitivity is regarded a key criterion for the choice of screening tools, their negative predictive value is usually better than the positive predictive value.

Let us calculate what typically happens when screening for a rare disease (frequency: 1 in 10,000 players) with the above considerations in mind (sensitivity of our screening tool: 97%; specificity: 90%, which is a quite good constellation): When 1,000,000 athletes are screened, the expected frequency of the disease is 100. With the given sensitivity, this means that 97 of the diseased players will be detected. However, due to the 90% specificity, 10% of the remaining 999,900 (= 99,990) players will be falsely diagnosed as having the disease. This means that only about 0.1% of the positive tests was correct, which gives us the (bad) positive predictive value. However, from the remaining 899,013 negative diagnoses, only 3 were wrong, which leads us to an almost perfect negative predictive value.

Not for all relevant diseases do we have screening tools with such an ideal combination of sensitivity and specificity. For example, the exercise electrocardiogram (ECG) for detecting coronary artery disease has a much worse sensitivity (around 50%) and specificity (around 75%), while the disease itself is more frequent. This obviously leads to a considerable number of missed diagnoses (and, thus, necessary additional screening examinations) and still a relevant number of falsely diagnosed diseases with all necessary follow-up investigations.

Precompetition screening for players competing in UEFA and FIFA tournaments are designed to identify diseases that might lead to fatal events during football match play or training. This approach is made with professional and other high-level players in mind and is intended to ensure the health of the players at all times and consequently protect the image of the sport and competition. Therefore, these regulations might exceed recommendations from medical societies that are formulated for the general athletic population. See the Medical Section at http://www.uefa.org for the most up-to-date UEFA Medical Regulations. FIFA precompetition medical examination regulations can also be obtained from the FIFA website.

## 9.3 Recommendations from Medical Societies

Recommendations from medical societies like the ESC (European Society of Cardiology,http://www.escardio.org/guidelines) or AHA/ACSM (American Heart Association/American College of Sports Medicine, http://circ.ahajournals.org/content/115/12/1643.full#sec-5) typically take into account the amount of money that has to be spent to prevent one player from a fatal (or otherwise detrimental) event, and thus may differ from those of a sports governing body. The differing costs for certain examinations between countries might play a role in such calculations. In this respect, echocardiography is crucial because it is frequently necessary to rule out or prove structural heart disease. Its higher costs in the U.S. partly explain the different guidelines between Europe and North America.

Whereas the European cardiologists recommend a resting ECG for all young athletes because of its low cost and its high negative predictive value, their American colleagues point to its unsatisfactory specificity and the expensive examinations which are to be done afterward in cases of a "positive" ECG. These costs, in contrast, would be much lower in many European countries.

## 9.4 Examinations during Pre-Competition Eligibility Screening

### 9.4.1 Types of Examination and Review of Results

For the purpose of screening in a symptomless footballer, the following examinations might be considered:

- Medical history.
- Physical examination.
- Resting ECG.
- Exercise ECG.
- Echocardiography.
- Laboratory values

If conducted, the points listed in **Table 9.1** are the key findings to be considered.

## 9.5 Examinations during Pretransfer Screening

The pretransfer screening is less defined and no mandatory requirements exist for which tests should be included. However, the doctor should always include a thorough history (+available information from other sources) and a physical examination. Other examinations are highly dependent on the gathered information during history and physical examination. In particular, the doctor should consider a targeted screening to identify issues related to previous injury and preconditions that could predict new injuries (e.g., ligament laxities). These should be searched for by appropriate imaging.

Due to the high costs involved with elite player transfers, the pressure on the screening doctor can often be extreme, and timescales can be very tight, particularly for imaging. It is therefore recommended that each team doctor has a clear idea in advance of the range of tests they would consider necessary for a transfer screening, including a menu of additional tests to account for the assessment of different types of previous injury.

The role of the doctor in pretransfer screening is not to make the decision on whether to sign the player or not, but to use the best available evaluation techniques and screening tools to provide the club staff with a prognosis for the player's future fitness to play, should the player be signed.

### 9.5.1 Common Problems with Eligibility Declarations

Besides an appropriate choice of examinations (which is usually decided by regulations from head organizations like UEFA or FIFA or the respective national bodies), several other issues associated with eligibility declarations might arise.

| Table 9.1 |
| --- |

**Key findings during precompetition eligibility screening**

| Examination type | Factors to consider |
| --- | --- |
| 1. Medical history | – known diseases and injuries<br>– family history of cardiovascular and other diseases<br>– early death in close relatives<br>– unexplained unconsciousness<br>– exercise-related problems (e.g., anginal and other pain, dyspnea, dizziness)<br>– earlier ineligibility declarations, surgery<br>– other stays in hospital, periods of absence from sport<br>– regular and spontaneous drug intake |
| 2. Physical examination | – among many other findings which are detected during a routine examination signs for Marfan's disease, auscultatory clicks, and murmurs with alterations due to position change, also large left-to-right blood pressure difference and abnormal peripheral pulses |
| 3. Resting ECG | – see new recommendations from the ESC and AHA (Drezner et al 2013) differentiating "normal" changes from dubious ones effectively |
| 4. Exercise ECG | – ST-segment changes indicative of ischemia, all kinds of exercise-induced rhythm disturbances; disappearance of dubious resting ECG findings indicates good prognosis<br>– Be aware of ethnic differences |
| 5. Echocardiography | – Experience is required to differentiate between an athlete's heart and other structural/pathological findings<br>– All kinds of cardiomyopathies should be screened for<br>– poor sensitivity for ischemic diseases<br>– difficult detection and frequently a case for pediatric cardiologists: abnormal course of coronary arteries<br>– Be aware of ethnic differences |
| 6. Laboratory values | – importance often overestimated<br>– mainly screening for manifest severe internal disease, e.g., diabetes, kidney disease<br>– Can also serve as basis for use of laboratory values as monitoring tools for training and competition stress (however, not purpose of the screening process itself) |

*Abbreviations: AHA, American Heart Association; ECG, electrocardiogram; ESC, European Society of Cardiology.*

Findings are not always 100% clear, which may preclude a simple yes-or-no decision. A good example for this might be cardiac changes compatible with the athlete's heart, but at the same time possibly indicative of structural heart disease. On the one hand, pathognomonic constellations of findings are not always complete in cases of manifest disease, but on the other, there is always the possibility that a disease is still in the process of development when the examination is performed. In such cases, statements about the likelihood of medical events might appear more appropriate than simple declarations of eligibility or ineligibility. Often a close follow-up evaluation would be made in cases of nonelite athletes, but this approach can be problematic in professional football players. Also, the time span of eligibility declarations is typically set at 1 year in professional football players. However, the development of relevant cardiac diseases might be faster in some cases. This can lead to the possibility of overlooking a developing disease.

All this possibly leads a team doctor to the question: Does a certain likelihood for a deterioration of complaints/diseases/injuries automatically lead to ineligibility of a player? If yes, it would be wise for the doctor to always stay on the safe side, but this approach could risk legal consequences where professional players would be banned from doing their business. And in such cases: Is a football player allowed to go to a number of other doctors until someone declares him eligible?

## Suggested Readings

[1] Basavarajaiah S, Boraita A, Whyte G, et al. Ethnic differences in left ventricular remodeling in highly-trained athletes relevance to differentiating physiologic left ventricular hypertrophy from hypertrophic cardiomyopathy. J Am Coll Cardiol. 2008; 51(23):2256–2262

[2] Bille K, Figueiras D, Schamasch P, et al. Sudden cardiac death in athletes: the Lausanne Recommendations. Eur J Cardiovasc Prev Rehabil. 2006; 13(6):859–875

[3] Bohm P, Ditzel R, Ditzel H, Urhausen A, Meyer T. Resting ECG findings in elite football players. J Sports Sci. 2013; 31(13):1475–1480

[4] Bohm P, Kästner A, Meyer T. Sudden cardiac death in football. J Sports Sci. 2013; 31 (13):1451–1459

[5] Chandra N, Papadakis M, Sharma S. Cardiac adaptation in athletes of black ethnicity: differentiating pathology from physiology. Heart. 2012; 98(16):1194–1200

[6] Chugh SS, Jui J, Gunson K, et al. Current burden of sudden cardiac death: multiple source

surveillance versus retrospective death certificate-based review in a large U.S. community. J Am Coll Cardiol. 2004; 44(6):1268–1275

[7] Corrado D, Basso C, Rizzoli G, Schiavon M, Thiene G. Does sports activity enhance the risk of sudden death in adolescents and young adults? J Am Coll Cardiol. 2003; 42(11):1959–1963

[8] Corrado D, Basso C, Schiavon M, Thiene G. Screening for hypertrophic cardiomyopathy in young athletes. N Engl J Med. 1998; 339 (6):364–369

[9] Corrado D, Pelliccia A, Heidbuchel H, et al. Section of Sports Cardiology, European Association of Cardiovascular Prevention and Rehabilitation,, Working Group of Myocardial and Pericardial Disease, European Society of Cardiology. Recommendations for interpretation of 12-lead electrocardiogram in the athlete. Eur Heart J. 2010; 31(2):243–259

[10] Drezner JA, Ackerman MJ, Anderson J, et al. Electrocardiographic interpretation in athletes: the 'Seattle criteria'. Br J Sports Med. 2013; 47(3):122–124

[11] Drezner JA, Ackerman MJ, Cannon BC, et al. Abnormal electrocardiographic findings in athletes: recognising changes suggestive of primary electrical disease. Br J Sports Med. 2013; 47(3):153–167

[12] Drezner JA, Ashley E, Baggish AL, et al. Abnormal electrocardiographic findings in athletes: recognising changes suggestive of cardiomyopathy. Br J Sports Med. 2013; 47(3):137–152

[13] Drezner JA, Fischbach P, Froelicher V, et al. Normal electrocardiographic findings: recognising physiological adaptations in athletes. Br J Sports Med. 2013; 47(3):125–136

[14] Eckart RE, Scoville SL, Campbell CL, et al. Sudden death in young adults: a 25-year review of autopsies in military recruits. Ann Intern Med. 2004; 141(11):829–834

[15] Harmon KG, Drezner JA, Wilson MG, Sharma S. Incidence of sudden cardiac death in athletes: a state-of-the-art review. Br J Sports Med. 2014; 48(15):1185–1192

[16] Koch S, Cassel M, Linné K, Mayer F, Scharhag J. ECG and echocardiographic findings in 10–15-year-old elite athletes. Eur J Prev Cardiol. 2014; 21(6):774–781

[17] Maron BJ, Haas TS, Doerer JJ, Thompson PD, Hodges JS. Comparison of U.S. and Italian experiences with sudden cardiac deaths in young competitive athletes and implications for preparticipation screening strategies. Am J Cardiol. 2009; 104(2):276–280

[18] Meister S, Faude O, Ammann T, Schnittker R, Meyer T. Indicators for high physical strain and overload in elite football players. Scand J Med Sci Sports. 2013; 23(2):156–163

[19] Meyer L, Stubbs B, Fahrenbruch C, et al. Incidence, causes, and survival trends from cardiovascular-related sudden cardiac arrest in children and young adults 0 to 35 years of age: a 30-year review. Circulation. 2012; 126 (11):1363–1372

[20] Meyer T, Meister S. Routine blood parameters in elite soccer players. Int J Sports Med. 2011; 32(11):875–881

[21] de Noronha SV, Sharma S, Papadakis M, Desai S, Whyte G, Sheppard MN. Aetiology of sudden cardiac death in athletes in the United Kingdom: a pathological study. Heart. 2009; 95 (17):1409–1414

[22] Pelliccia A, Maron BJ, Culasso F, et al. Clinical significance of abnormal electrocardiographic patterns in trained athletes. Circulation. 2000; 102(3):278–284

[23] Scharhag J, Löllgen H, Kindermann W. Competitive sports and the heart: benefit or risk? Dtsch Arztebl Int. 2013; 110(1–2):14–23, quiz 24, e1–e2

[24] Schmied C, Borjesson M. Sudden cardiac death in athletes. J Intern Med. 2014; 275(2):93–103

[25] Schmied C, Di Paolo FM, Zerguini AY, Dvorak J, Pelliccia A. Screening athletes for cardiovascular disease in Africa: a challenging experience. Br J Sports Med. 2013; 47(9):579–584

[26] Schmied C, Zerguini Y, Junge A, et al. Cardiac findings in the precompetition medical assessment of football players participating in the 2009 African Under-17 Championships in Algeria. Br J Sports Med. 2009; 43 (9):716–721

[27] Suárez-Mier MP, Aguilera B, Mosquera RM, Sánchez-de-León MS. Pathology of sudden death during recreational sports in Spain. Forensic Sci Int. 2013; 226(1–3):188–196

[28] Thünenkötter T, Schmied C, Grimm K, Dvorak J, Kindermann W. Precompetition cardiac assessment of football players participating in the 2006 FIFA World Cup Germany. Clin J Sport Med. 2009; 19(4):322–325

[29] Weiner RB, Hutter AM, Wang F, et al. Performance of the 2010 European Society of Cardiology criteria for ECG interpretation in athletes. Heart. 2011; 97(19):1573–1577

9

# Appendix 1

## The Drill Framework

## A1.1 Introduction

This framework is a simple set of drills which aims to touch on all the various functional movement patterns a player will require to return to training. All the drills can be adapted or modified as required, but as with any drill, the important thing is to recognize what the drills are asking the player to do and why they are being used.

In **Fig. A1.1**, the various types of movement demands necessary for normal football function are identified. These demands include running-based patterns (yellow), other functional movement patterns (green), ball work (red), goalkeeper work (blue), and there is a blank space. This blank space represents other aspects you wish to include that have not been identified or that may be specific to the player. All of these functional demands can be addressed using football function to drive the progression. Some you will be more focused on due to the pathology you are dealing with, but all are part of playing football, which is basis of this framework.

## A1.2 Framework Diagram

Further diagrams have been generated with a simple software package, which can be useful to store and create sessions, and to reprint as required. Even if you simply draw your session and drills on a piece of paper, it will always be more effective and productive if you have invested time in planning the session in advance. Planning makes sure you include the correct drills, know what equipment you need, and can also be a reference during the session to know what you are doing next.

Importantly your session plan is a guide and needs to be flexible. Sometimes you may change the order of what you do, modify a drill because the player is not comfortable doing a certain movement, or after the first set you may decide to remove a particular movement for the second repetition. You may skip a drill because you decide after the session has started that the player is moving well enough and can move on having done the drill well on previous days. You may decide to repeat a drill more times than you planned for because you think that the player will benefit from the repetition and is not ready to progress. Having planned well, the key is to watch the player and reflect on the quality of the player's performance and react to what you see.

Eventually you will know your drills well enough that you can just list the drill title in your plan and know what the drill is without the diagram. Good preparation will allow you to apply a consistent approach.

### A1.2.1 Diagram Key

This diagram shows the key to the content of each of the drills explained in this section (**Fig. A1.2**). Note (1) the different colored lines for different movement intensities and (2) the different types of lines which

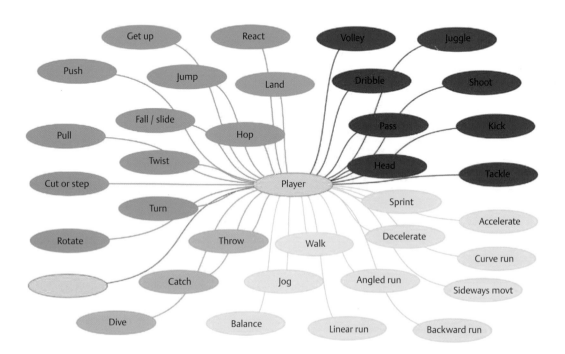

**Fig. A1.1**    The functional movement demands of football.

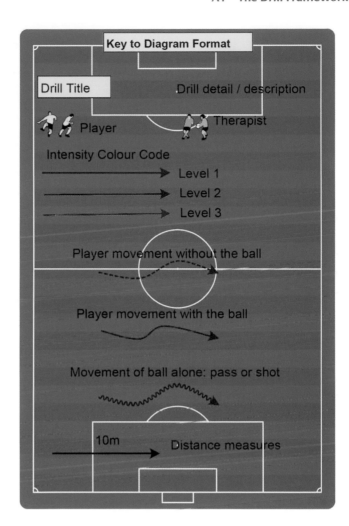

**Fig. A1.2**   Diagram key.

show whether the player is moving with the ball, without the ball, or if the ball is moving alone, i.e., a pass. Note also that players are identified in a yellow shirt and the therapist, which could be any member of the medical department, is identified in a blue shirt.

### A1.2.2  Basic Equipment Requirements

This diagram shows the basic equipment required for this framework (**Fig. A1.3**). Most drills can be performed with this basic set of equipment, but if you do not have this equipment, simply adapt. Poles can be replaced with cones. Having another staff member with you can replace the bounce board. Players can move around a cluster of cones rather than a hoop.

### A1.2.3  The Warm-Up

This diagram lists the basic sequence of activities that can be included in a warm-up (**Fig. A1.4**). There are many ways to warm-up, and your session design

is up to you. The method chosen may be influenced by the weather, your equipment, the player, or the stage of progression and other variables such as the session about to be undertaken. For example, due to cold weather conditions, you may choose to start the warm-up inside, use a bike instead of a run to start, and do the static stretches indoors. That way when you get outside, the player is already warm and can begin the session without the need for static stretching, for example.

### A1.2.4  Light Multidirectional Movements

This diagram shows an example of how to structure the multidirectional warm-up movements you may wish to perform in the warm-up (**Fig. A1.5**). Try to get in the habit of addressing all joints and muscle groups. One method you could use is to start with movements of the hips and back and then target joints and muscles one at a time in a logical progression from the back to the feet, making sure you

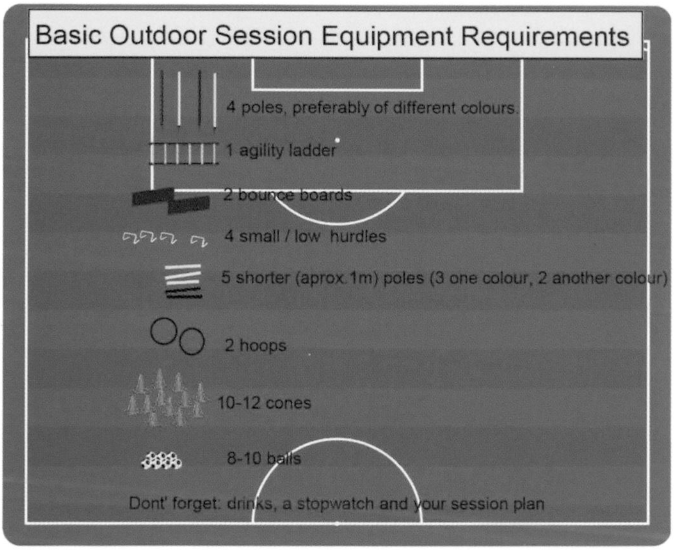

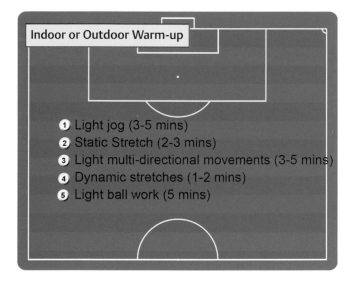

Fig. A1.3   Basic equipment requirements.

Fig. A1.4   The warm-up.

stimulate all areas. There are lots of different movement patterns, but having a system makes sure you perform at least one pattern for each area of the body. In this example provided, the therapist simply demonstrates what the player is to do between the cones.

### A1.2.5 Light Ball Work

This diagram gives an example of some light ball-work routines you can use in the warm-up (**Fig. A1.6**). Here you start with the player on the spot (1) and do some touches of the ball. The player does some passes on the spot (2), and then moves side to side or forward and back to pass the ball (3). Use any variation of movement you like to get the player to

touch the ball, pass the ball, and move to or with the ball.

### A1.2.6 Multidirectional Circuits

**Table A1.1** shows what a "normal dose" of drills 7, 8, and 9 might be and how these drills might be progressed using the variables discussed earlier.

Having seen the player perform all basic multidirectional movement patterns in isolation in the warm-up, and having done some basic passing in the warm-up, you can now introduce a more complex drill where the player combines these movements with a pass in a more structured way. These drills are designed to get the player to move side to side, forward and back, turn in each direction, and

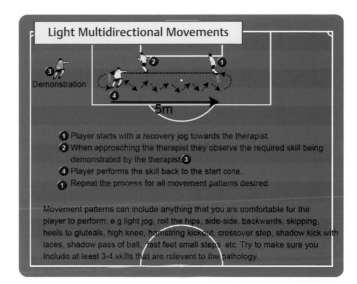

**Fig. A1.5**  Light multidirectional movements.

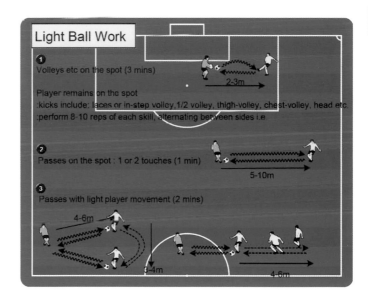

**Fig. A1.6**  Light ball work.

stimulate more precise motor control and vertical body movements. Importantly in the first circuit (**Fig. A1.7**), the player moves without the ball so he/she can concentrate on a quality movement pattern. You can get the player to move in the direction and manner you want by structuring your equipment accordingly. Your imagination is your only limitation on the skills they perform. Aim to include five to six skill paths in this type of drill, as it requires this many skills to stimulate all the different movement patterns. It normally takes the player approximately 60 to 90 seconds to complete this drill at level 1 intensity in this format. Time though is not important in the early stages, so just get the player to focus on quality of his/her movement.

If you feel you need to introduce these movements more carefully, there is no reason why you could not do each skill pathway in isolation a few times before combining them into a circuit. You may do the isolated paths one day and combine them the next or you could do them in isolation first and then do them in the circuit in the same session.

These drills will act to further warm up the player, and in later stages can be used for developing a volume of work by doing more sets, by including more skill stations in the path or by working to time. In that case, you could use time to govern how long the player works, where he/she simply continues through the circuit and goes back to the start and continues until the time has elapsed.

| Table A1.1 | |
|---|---|
| **"Normal dose" of drills 7, 8, and 9** | |
| **Fig. A1.7, Fig. A1.8, Fig. A1.9**<br>**Normal drill dosage** | **2–3 sets each lasting 60–90 s** |
| Drill variation and progression options | |
| Intensity | To progress these drills using intensity, use an increase in intensity level when moving away from the therapist (e.g., Level 2) and then a lower intensity to facilitate a degree of recovery as the player moves back toward the therapist (e.g., Level 1). See **Fig. A1.8**. |
| Space | To progress these drills using space, increase the distances that a player runs away from the therapist to turn around the cone. Bigger space to cover will mean the player covers more distance and works for a longer time if you keep the same number of pathways. |
| Time/volume | To progress this drill using time or volume, the number of sets can increase (volume) or the number of skill pathways and therefore the time taken to complete the drill can be increased. |
| Movement | To progress this drill via the type of movement, the skills, for example, can be progressed using more poles for the slalom path, use bigger hurdles that will require higher leg movements, use more complex foot movement combinations through the ladder, movement backward through the poles, etc. |
| Complexity | To progress this drill though content complexity, you could include a pass at either end of the skill pathway if you included a bounce board or had another therapist to use. You could include two to three passes at each end or have two different skills along the same path. |
| Reaction | N/A: For these drills, progression is better achieved using other variables. |

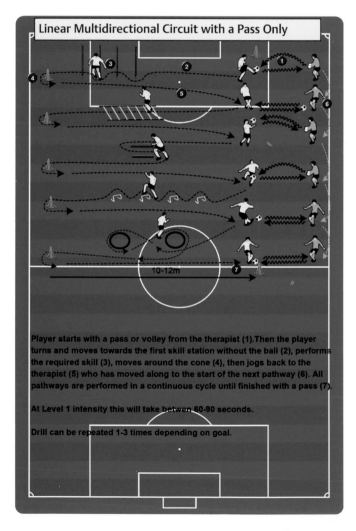

**Linear Multidirectional Circuit with a Pass Only**

10–12m

Player starts with a pass or volley from the therapist (1).Then the player turns and moves towards the first skill station without the ball (2), performs the required skill (3), moves around the cone (4), then jogs back to the therapist (5) who has moved along to the start of the next pathway (6). All pathways are performed in a continuous cycle until finished with a pass (7).

At Level 1 intensity this will take between 60-90 seconds.

Drill can be repeated 1-3 times depending on goal.

**Fig. A1.7**   Linear multidirectional circuit with a pass.

The design and structure of your circuit can vary. In **Fig. A1.8**, the same multidirectional circuit format is delivered in a fan shape rather than a linear format. Variation of the drill layout can be useful to give some variety for a player, particularly one who will do several sessions. For example, a player who is being rehabilitated for an anterior cruciate ligament reconstruction will do this type of drill many times. For this type of player, you may need to regularly modify the way the drill looks to avoid boredom. Use different equipment and different shapes to create a variety of drills.

As mentioned earlier, variety is good, but familiarity is also good, particularly when you are progressing a drill in some way. For example in **Fig. A1.9**, the same fan circuit is progressed by getting the player to work at a level 2 intensity when moving away from the therapist, and then return (recovering) to the therapist at a level 1 intensity. When progressing an aspect of function, a player will value a familiar drill, so he/she does not need to think about what to do skill wise, but rather can concentrate on the change, in this case the intensity.

### A1.2.7  Multidirectional Circuit with the Ball

Now that the player has performed multidirectional movements with confidence and quality *without* the ball, they can progress by moving *with* the ball

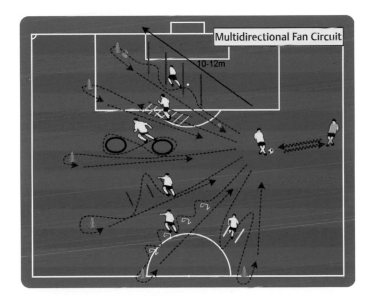

**Fig. A1.8**  Fan-shaped multidirectional circuit with a pass.

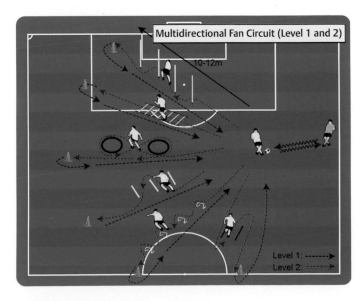

**Fig. A1.9**  Fan-shaped multidirectional circuit with a pass (Level 1 and 2 intensity).

(**Fig. A1.10**). When a player moves with the ball, he/she needs to perform more corrective and reactive movements to adapt to the movement of the ball and adjust foot position to manipulate the ball. These movement adjustments place increased demand on the player (**Table A1.2**).

## A1.2.8 Passing and Kicking

This framework aims to get the player starting to touch the ball as soon as possible (**Fig. A1.11**). For some injuries, this might mean starting to kick the ball with the noninjured leg on the spot and then beginning light touches with the injured leg. The pathology will influence how fast you can introduce passing and kicking, but as always, if you start at the most basic level and progress step by step you should not have any concerns. For example, with a thigh muscle injury, risk may be associated with either strong or rapid tension that might be generated with kicking the ball. If,

however, the player can do resisted muscle activation on the treatment couch or has been kicking, for example, in a swimming pool against the drag of the water, then there should be no reason to not start light touches of the ball. Sometimes you may choose to start passing with a soft ball that has less mass and therefore does not require the muscle to work as hard (e.g., a partially inflated volleyball). This can start a kicking progression when there is some risk associated with the injury type and can help the player build confidence before they progress to the normal ball.

Passing can be included as part of a more complex drill, but sometimes it is useful to set aside time between drills to complete 10 to 15 passes in a controlled fashion, so you know they are performing the kick or pass with quality over the distance you want without any discomfort. You may do 3 to 4 specific sets of 10 to 15 passes in a session, all at the same level or you may progress the passing as you feel

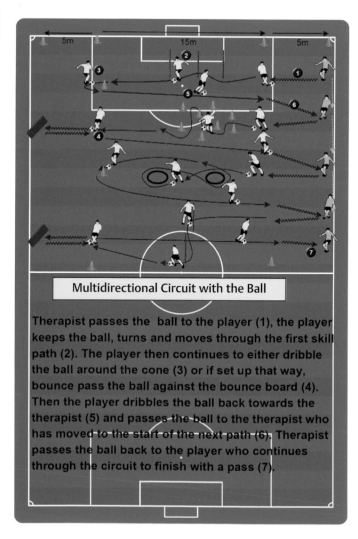

**Multidirectional Circuit with the Ball**

Therapist passes the ball to the player (1), the player keeps the ball, turns and moves through the first skill path (2). The player then continues to either dribble the ball around the cone (3) or if set up that way, bounce pass the ball against the bounce board (4). Then the player dribbles the ball back towards the therapist (5) and passes the ball to the therapist who has moved to the start of the next path (6). Therapist passes the ball back to the player who continues through the circuit to finish with a pass (7).

**Fig. A1.10**  Multidirectional circuit with the ball.

| Table A1.2 |
|---|

**Multidirectional circuit with the ball**

| Fig. A1.10:<br>Normal drill dosage | Two to three sets each lasting 60–90 seconds each |
|---|---|
| | Drill variation and progression options |
| Intensity | To progress this drill using intensity, use an increase in intensity level when moving away from the therapist (e.g., Level 2 or 3) and then a lower intensity to recover as the player moves back toward the therapist (e.g., Level 1). |
| Space | To progress this drill using space, increase the distances that a player moves with the ball away from the therapist. Bigger space to cover will mean the player covers more distance and therefore works for longer. |
| Time/volume | To progress this drill using volume, the number of sets can increase or the number of skill pathways can be increased. |
| Movement | To progress this drill via the type of movement, the skills can be progressed via changing the type of task required, for example, by using more poles to dribble through or by using more cones to randomly dribble past. |
| Complexity | To progress this drill though content complexity, you could include a pass at either end of the skill pathway or in the middle of a pathway off a bounce board. You could also include a small goal at the end of a pathway with a bounce board for the player to pass/shoot into and then return back to the therapist without a ball, keeping the ball passed them as they continue. You could also throw or bounce the ball to the player so they need to control it before they move through a skill pathway. |
| Reaction | N/A |

A1

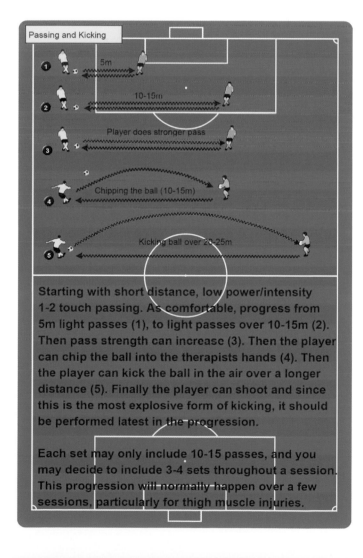

**Fig. A1.11**   Passing and kicking.

suitable. By introducing passing early, you allow yourself longer to progress this skill, i.e., if you wait until halfway through your rehab to introduce passing, then you will need to progress it quickly, whereas if you start early, you can take smaller, more regular steps. Remember that controlled functional stressing of the muscle and injured area will also facilitate more functional tissue healing, which could result in a better outcome (**Table A1.3**).

### A1.2.9 Basic Strength, Power, and Proprioceptive Exercises

This framework has functional movement as the main focus for the rehabilitation progression (**Fig. A1.12**). With many injuries, you may also

want to supplement some strength, power, or proprioceptive work specific to the pathology. These additional activities can be performed on the pitch or indoors. You may choose to include them as part of a functional session or perform them separately at a different time. It is important to be conscious of the volume and dosage of exercises you are getting the injured player to perform. It is very easy to do too much by, for example, doing a session on grass and a session in the gym on the same day. You may choose to include specific strength exercise for muscle injuries such as hamstring injuries, for example, so that you are confident that the pathology is rehabilitated thoroughly. These additional exercises will be in the form of either manually resisted

| Table A1.3 | |
|---|---|
| **Passing and kicking** | |
| **Fig. A1.11:** Normal drill dosage | **Three to four sets of 10–15 passes/kicks spread out through a session** |
| Drill variation and progression options | |
| Intensity | To modify this drill using intensity, you can start with a soft ball, or to progress you can increase the strength or power of the pass or kick. |
| Space | To progress this drill using space, you can increase the distance the player needs to kick over, which will require a pass or kick with greater strength. |
| Volume | To progress this drill using volume, the number of sets and repetitions can increase. Remember, however, that in a game a player never performs 20 kicks in a row in close succession, so normally 10–15 kicks in a set is sufficient. Make sure you alternate between legs during a set so you do not overload the leg unnecessarily. |
| Movement | To progress this drill via the type of movement, you could pass the ball into space that the player needs to move to, and then you can move to another position where they need to pass to you. |
| Complexity | To progress this drill though content complexity, you could have the pass as part of a more complex drill; include a longer ball or a shot at the end of a drill. You should ensure that the passing level you are asking them to perform in the more complex drill has been performed in isolation so there will be no issue with confidence. |
| Reaction | To progress this drill using reaction, you can place a few different colored target such as cones or poles and when you pass the ball to the player, you call a color. The player then needs to control the ball and pass with accuracy to the selected target. |

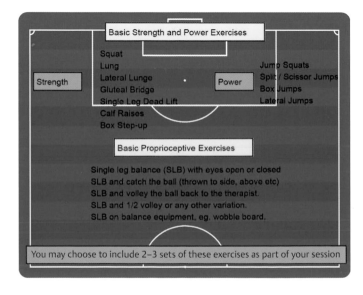

**Fig. A1.12** Basic strength, power, and proprioceptive exercises.

exercise on the treatment couch, isokinetic strengthening exercises using an isokinetic device, or exercises in the gym.

Proprioceptive exercises for joint-based injuries such as ankle sprains may be useful, using soft cushion mats, wobble boards, BOSUs, and mini-trampolines for challenging balance. Sometimes these activities will be used as part of a warm-up when the player is familiar and comfortable doing the exercise in question, but they can also occur as part of a session, being included between drills.

The approach in using these exercises should be consistent with the overall philosophy, in that you always start at the most basic level and progress as comfortable. For example, if you had a player with a rectus femoris muscle injury, you would not start with dynamic split jumps as this is a power-based exercise, which will challenge the muscle at a high level. A more logical progression example for this exercise is represented below, and could be progressed over several sessions.

— **Step 1:** Therapist is comfortable the player can stretch into the range of motion to be used, e.g., player can do a static quadriceps stretch pain free.
— **Step 2:** Player positions feet in lunge position and performs one set or eight repetitions of a static lunge where foot position does not change. Exercise is repeated for each leg, i.e., reverse leg positions. This single set can be repeated three times at once or spread out during the session between drills.
— **Step 3:** Player starts with feet together and then steps forward into and then back out of a lunge position, alternating each rep between each leg. Player does one set of eight repetitions per leg

and repeats this set three times throughout a session.
— **Step 4:** Same as step 3 but with more a dynamic push movement to get back out of the lunge position.
— **Step 5:** Player starts in a lunge step position and then jumps up in the air and while in the air, the feet positions change so that they land in the reverse position. Then this movement is repeated for four to eight jumps.
— **Step 6:** Player performs six split jumps (three per side) with a quick transition between each jump. Two to three sets can be performed throughout a session.

## A1.2.10 Reaction: Four Poles

This sequence of diagrams provides a good example of how a basic drill can be adjusted in a minor way to provide a different challenge for the player. The same concept can be applied to most drills, so it is useful to understand how the small changes shown change the nature and demands of the drill.

**Fig. A1.13** shows the most basic version of the four-pole drill. Here the therapist passes a ball to the player who is standing in the middle of the four poles. The player passes the ball back to the therapist and then moves without the ball toward a pole of his/her choice, touches the pole, and then returns to the middle of the square to receive another pass. The process is repeated until eight touches have occurred. Here the player is in control of the direction of movement, and they can move in any sequence they choose as long as they touch each pole twice over the set. This drill can be introduced early in a rehab progression as it can be performed at a

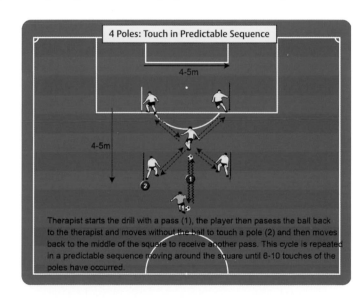

**Fig. A1.13** Four poles with a predictable touch.

low intensity, in a predictable manner and it is a very functional and specific movement pattern for a footballer.

**Fig. A1.14** is a progression from **Fig. A1.13** as it changes the drill by requiring the player to move *around* the pole rather than just touch it. This makes the drill a little more complex in terms of movement and it requires the player to turn in all directions. The way the player turns around the pole could also be modified, e.g., curving around the pole, moving around the pole keeping shoulders and hips square to the therapist, or the player could move around the front of the pole first or go around the back of the pole first.

**Fig. A1.15** shows the introduction to the *reaction* component of the drill sequence. Here the player is performing the same movement as in **Fig. A1.13**, but now the poles are marked in some way so that they each have a different color. As the therapist passes the ball, he/she calls a color that the player must move to and touch after he passes the ball back to the therapist. The therapist calls colors at random to make the player react and move in random directions. The therapist might call the same color in a row, for example, which will require a reactive movement from the player that they might not have expected. This drill therefore starts to introduce unpredictable movements, requires the player to be

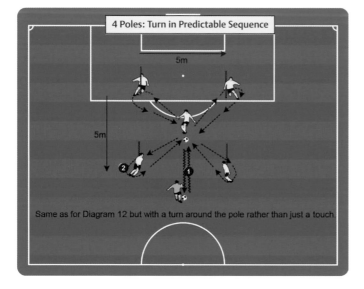

**Fig. A1.14**  Four poles with a predictable turn.

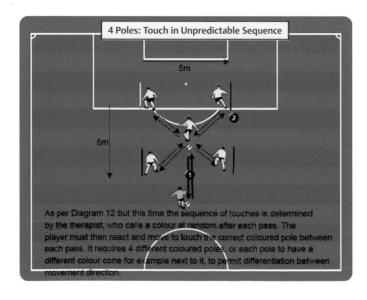

**Fig. A1.15**  Four poles with an unpredictable touch.

aware of the space around him/her, and is therefore a reactive progression of function, as opposed to the drill in **Fig. A1.13** where the player was in control of movement direction.

**Fig. A1.16** then applies an unpredictable sequence to the four-pole drill where the player must move around the pole (**Table A1.4**).

## A1.2.11  Speed, Agility, and Quickness

Football is a game that requires random movements in numerous different patterns at a high intensity (**Fig. A1.17**). Speed, Agility, and Quickness (SAQ)

drills help introduce many different patterns of movement, help develop motor coordination, confidence in reactive agility movements, and also act to improve the "sharpness" of a player. As always, they should be introduced at "Level 1" intensity and then progressed in intensity and complexity as quality and confidence progress. They can then also be combined with other skills to create more complex combination drills.

As the name suggests, these drills aim to get players to perform fast, agile movements at speed. The movements are governed by the path that is set out using

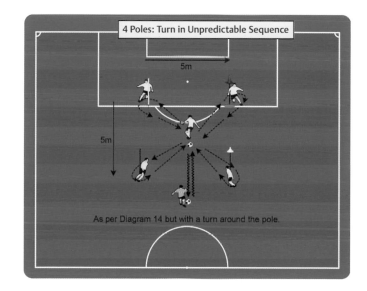

**Fig. A1.16**  Four poles with an unpredictable turn.

| A1 |

**Table A1.4**

| Reaction: four poles | |
| --- | --- |
| **Fig. A1.13, Fig. A1.14, Fig. A1.15, Fig. A1.16: Normal drill dosage** | **Three to four sets of 6–10 touches or turns** |
| Drill variation and progression options | |
| Intensity | To progress this drill using intensity, you can ask the player to work at level 1.5, 2, or 3 intensity. |
| Space | To progress this drill using space, you can make the square smaller, e.g., 3-m square, and the player has to move at a level 2 intensity. This will place a greater demand on the muscles due to the quick concentric/eccentric start/stop work required. If you open the space up to 6-m square, then the player has a longer space to accelerate and decelerate, so this is another way to progress the drill. |
| Time/volume | To progress this drill using volume, the number of sets and repetitions can increase. Worthy of note though is that four sets of high-intensity movements with six to eight repetitions is quite tiring and a significant load, so this is not the best method of progressing this drill unless it is done with that goal in mind. |
| Movement | To progress this drill via type of movement, you can use the touch or turn variation. You could also call the color and also call to "touch" or "turn," so the player has to think about not only the color, but also what movement is required, e.g., "red, touch." |
| Complexity | To progress this drill though content complexity, you could ask the player to keep the ball and move around the pole with the ball. You could also ask the player to half volley or head the ball, depending on your delivery of the ball to them. You could also position more than four poles. |
| Reaction | To progress this drill using reaction, you use the color variation and by delaying the call of the color until just as the player passes the ball, you require a quicker reaction. You can also make sure the pass is on its way to the player as they touch or turn around the pole so that they need to react to the ball faster as they return to the center of the space. |

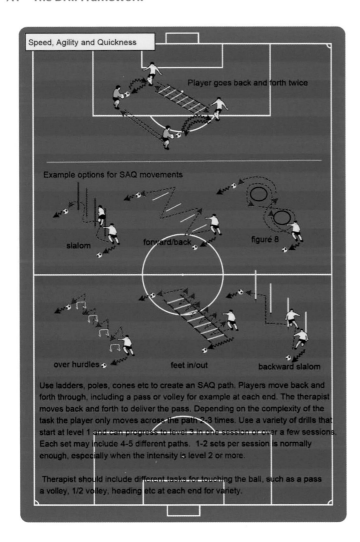

**Fig. A1.17**   Speed, agility, and quickness.

your available equipment (e.g., cones or poles). Players are asked to move though the path with a specific movement pattern which will often require a basic demonstration from the therapist. Any movement pattern can be developed that you feel is useful for the player's rehabilitation. When introducing these drills, include some patterns that challenge the pathology you are rehabilitating and some that are not directly challenging the pathology. For example, for a hamstring injury, movements with linear acceleration and deceleration are particularly challenging, so these sorts of patterns can be combined with paths that require lateral movements (**Table A1.5**).

## A1.2.12  Acceleration and Deceleration
It is essential for a player to be able to accelerate and decelerate. This skill is also something that has a direct relationship with muscle injuries such as thigh muscle strains, which account for a large proportion of time-loss injuries in football.

**Fig. A1.18** shows a basic drill that can be used to develop this capacity. Very low intensity acceleration will have already been performed in early drills such as in the multidirectional movement drills performed earlier in the progression, so normally by the time you think about introducing these skills, you will have already started the progression. The player starts at the first cone and accelerates forward until they have covered about 50% of the distance to the finish pole. At this point, the player starts to decelerate. There is logic in the thought that you should not focus on acceleration until you can also decelerate, so by starting with 50% of the distance accelerating and then using the other 50% to decelerate the player should be safe.

For this drill, it is better to identify the intensity you desire using a percentage effort system, as it will permit you more stages to progress through than just the Level 1 to 3 system. For example, start with the player accelerating at "50% effort," and get them

| Table A1.5 | |
| --- | --- |
| **Speed, agility, and quickness** | |
| **Fig. A1.17: Normal drill dosage** | One to two sets each of five to six skill pathways |
| Drill variation and progression options | |
| Intensity | To progress this drill using intensity, you can ask the player to work at level 1.5, 2, or level 3 intensity. |
| Space | To progress this drill using space in different ways, either encourage tighter movements at a higher intensity, which will place a high load on the muscles, or place equipment over a bigger space, which will make the player work harder due to distance. |
| Volume | To progress this drill using volume, the number of sets and repetitions can increase. As performance quality and intensity increase, you may choose to make the volume smaller and do less repetitions in a set or you may need to give greater recovery time between drills. |
| Movement | To progress this drill via the type of movement, you can use combinations of movement by putting two skills together. |
| Complexity | To progress this drill though content complexity, you could ask the player to keep the ball and move around the pole with the ball, for example. You could also ask the player to half volley or head the ball, depending on your delivery of the ball to them. |
| Reaction | To progress this drill using reaction, you can use the color variation or you can include a pass or volley at random during the path. |

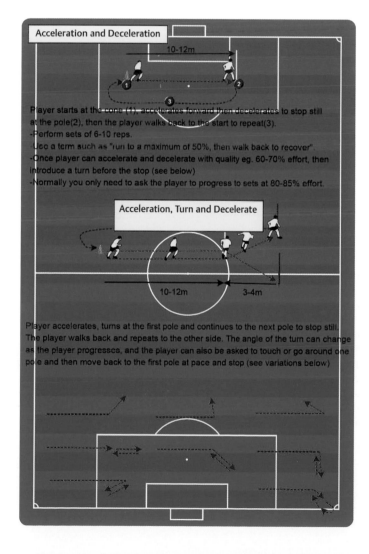

**Acceleration and Deceleration**

10-12m

Player starts at the cone (1), accelerates forward then decelerates to stop still at the pole(2), then the player walks back to the start to repeat(3).
-Perform sets of 6-10 reps.
-Use a term such as "run to a maximum of 50%, then walk back to recover".
-Once player can accelerate and decelerate with quality eg. 60-70% effort, then introduce a turn before the stop (see below)
-Normally you only need to ask the player to progress to sets at 80-85% effort.

**Acceleration, Turn and Decelerate**

10-12m          3-4m

Player accelerates, turns at the first pole and continues to the next pole to stop still. The player walks back and repeats to the other side. The angle of the turn can change as the player progresses, and the player can also be asked to touch or go around one pole and then move back to the first pole at pace and stop (see variations below)

**Fig. A1.18**   Acceleration and deceleration.

to perform six to eight runs at this percentage. In the first session, you may do two to three sets of this intensity for the player to become familiar. If however the pathology is not something that gives you concern about progressing the muscle load, e.g., an ankle sprain, then after the first set of six accelerations you may ask the player to accelerate at 60%. Once you start this progression, you should also ask the player to accelerate for a longer part of the distance and then decelerate. For example, you can stand in the middle of the distance between the start cone and finish pole and ask the player to accelerate until he/she is next to you, and then start decelerating. As you want to reduce the distance of the deceleration, which increases the load on muscles, you can take a step toward the finish pole to guide the player. Make sure in these early drills that the player knows to stop still at the finish pole. Just slowing down does not stress the muscle the same way as stopping still, and in a match being able to stop still and change direction is an essential skill.

Once you are comfortable that that player can perform the drill at 60 to 70%, you can introduce a turn in the drill. Players often need to change direction while running at pace, so this drill will develop this capacity. By using two more poles that are placed outside the original finish pole, you can direct the player to accelerate straight ahead, turn at the first pole, and then continue to the next pole to stop. By placing a pole on each side in the same pattern and alternating the sides that the player turns toward, you can ensure the challenge is undertaken for both directions. You can progress this drill by making the angle of direction change greater. The greater the change in direction and therefore change in momentum of the player, the greater the demand on the muscles. Therefore, the most challenging will be accelerating, decelerating, and then accelerating back in the direction they came from. **Fig. A1.18** shows examples of different variations that can be developed in conjunction with progression of intensity. It is not recommended to ask a player to perform these drills at 100%. Aim for 85% and often they will work harder anyway. Remember that returning to training is the last stage of rehab and so there will be some things the player does not do until they are back in training for a few sessions. Players need to understand this too, and be smart about how they settle back into the training environment (**Table A1.6**).

### A1.2.13 Combination Drill

**Fig. A1.19** is a good example of combining different skills you will have done in their basic forms in isolation earlier in the rehabilitation, to create a more functional combination drill. This drill combines a pass, which could also be a volley, a head of the ball, or anything you select; then, the player moves through an SAQ pathway (which again could be any skill the player has completed previously), accelerates, decelerates to turn, and then accelerates and decelerates again. This sort of drill will be performed later in the rehab progression when the player has shown that he/she is comfortable and confident to deliver any movement pattern. If a player can perform this sort of drill with quality and intensity, then you will know they

| Table A1.6 | |
|---|---|
| **Acceleration and deceleration** | |
| **Fig. A1.18:** Normal drill dosage | **Two to three sets of 6–10 runs** |
| Drill variation and progression options | |
| Intensity | To progress this drill using intensity, you can ask the player to work at 50, 60, 75%, etc., of their maximum intensity. |
| Space | To progress this drill using space, you can make the distance of the first acceleration longer. A longer run gives greater distance to speed up and therefore will require greater effort to slow down. A distance of 10–12 m should be sufficient to get a strong acceleration. At lengths of less than 10 m, players often do not have enough distance to build up a strong acceleration. Similarly, more than 15 m is not really necessary for this drill. |
| Volume | To progress this drill using volume, the number of sets and repetitions can increase, but like other drills, as the *quality* increases you need to either give longer rest periods or do less repetitions. When a player is performing this drill at 85–90%, you should normally only get them to do a one to two set of four to six repetitions. |
| Movement | To progress this drill via the type of movement, you change the angle of the turn. The greater the change in direction and therefore momentum, the greater the load. You could also get the player to turn around the pole and not just stop at it or touch it. |
| Complexity | This drill is focused on acceleration and deceleration, and by making it too complex, you can detract from the quality of the acceleration. Therefore, the other variables such as volume, space, etc., offer better methods of progression. |
| Reaction | To progress this drill using reaction, you use different colored poles to turn toward. When the player approaches the first pole, the therapist can call a color to determine the direction they need to move off in. |

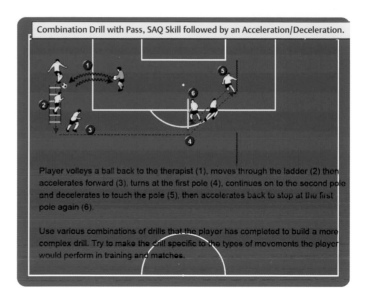

Combination Drill with Pass, SAQ Skill followed by an Acceleration/Deceleration.

Player volleys a ball back to the therapist (1), moves through the ladder (2) then accelerates forward (3), turns at the first pole (4), continues on to the second pole and decelerates to touch the pole (5), then accelerates back to stop at the first pole again (6).

Use various combinations of drills that the player has completed to build a more complex drill. Try to make the drill specific to the types of movements the player would perform in training and matches.

**Fig. A1.19**   Combination drill.

are not far from a training environment with respect to their movements.

To progress this drill, modify the various drill building blocks in the same way you would when you performed the drill in isolation. It is only your imagination that will limit you here, but be careful not to make the drill so complex that the player cannot give you quality because he/she is trying to remember what to do.

This also raises an important point. Part of the rehab process is to make sure the player experiences success or that they can see what they have done has been done correctly. If you make a drill so complex or difficult that the player cannot complete it successfully, you are setting them up to fail, which is counterproductive. The challenge of a drill needs to match the player's stage of recovery and skill level and their capacity to follow the instructions. For example, early in the rehab progression you may use a drill where the player has to finish the drill with a pass of the ball between two poles that are 1 m apart, from a distance of 10 m.

Most players could experience some good success with this drill. If late in the rehab progression, however, when you want to reinforce to the player that they are "almost back," if you make it almost impossible for the player to succeed (e.g., shoot the ball through a small hoop you have hanging from a goal from 20 m), then it is unlikely they will succeed several times. There is a big psychological component to rehab and the player needs to feel they are improving; hence, you should ensure that they can perform functional movements with quality, and experience success in the drills you design for them.

## A1.2.14  Runs

Being able to run is an integral part of playing football. It is essential before a player returns to training that they can run without pain over a distance they might be required to run in training, that they can run with good intensity, and that their physical condition is such that one run does not completely fatigue them. For these reasons, look to include runs in sessions from an early stage. Most players find doing lots of long runs boring. So try to include sets of runs throughout a session, and progress the nature of the runs as appropriate. Performing runs as part of a session progression is also useful as a method of physical conditioning for the player (**Fig. A1.20**).

As per the philosophy, start with runs at a low intensity over a longer distance. Players can be asked to run the full length of the pitch at low intensity and then walk the return length. Often though for most injuries, you can start with a light run (e.g., 40% effort) running half the length of the pitch and then walk or jog slowly for the second half of the pitch. Intensity can progress through increasing the percentage effort, increasing the number of runs in a set, or by asking the player to jog the recovery part of the drill at a higher intensity than previously performed. As the intensity increases, the distance covered can reduce. Importantly, the other drills included in this framework require runs of short distance and high intensity, so you normally will not need to do runs shorter than the distance from the halfway line to the top of the 18-yard box.

Look to include two to three sets of four to eight runs in a session for a player that has been out of training for a few weeks as these runs will

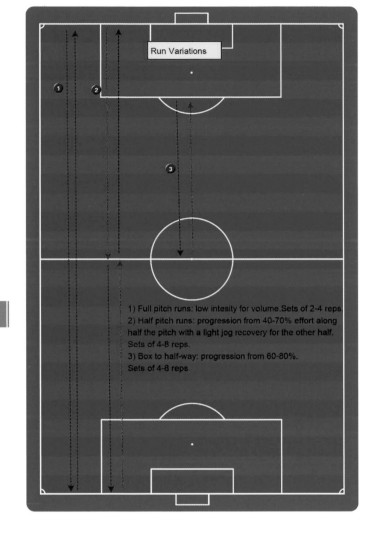

**Run Variations**

1) Full pitch runs: low intesity for volume.Sets of 2-4 reps.
2) Half pitch runs: progression from 40-70% effort along half the pitch with a light jog recovery for the other half. Sets of 4-8 reps.
3) Box to half-way: progression from 60-80%. Sets of 4-8 reps

**Fig. A1.20**   Runs.

develop some conditioning of the player so that they can better cope with training in terms of conditioning. If a player is only out of training for a short period, however, such as a few days, then the purpose of doing the runs is more to reassure both you and the player that they can complete these runs without difficulty. Under these circumstances, you only need to complete one set in a session as they will not have deconditioned much, and the goal of the drill is different from when you are rehabilitating a player after a long-term injury (**Table A1.7**).

### A1.2.15 Position-Specific Drills
The start of this section of the chapter recommended looking at the type of function a player is required to perform in normal training or match play, and to use that as a target for the rehab to work toward. Position-specific drills are the final drills that the rehabilitation progression culminates in, where the player works at a moderate to high intensity, doing combinations of skills and movements that they may do in a match in an intense period of play. They should be specific to the normal playing position of the player and will therefore differ for different players. These are drills that should prove to both you and the player that they can be reintroduced into the training environment confidently. They should have components that challenge the player across the different design variables, i.e., they should be high-intensity drills and contain dynamic, reactive, and complex movement patterns.

The drills in **Fig. A1.21** and **Fig. A1.22** show examples for a defending and attacking player, respectively. They are one example of a possible drill configuration, but by simply watching video footage of a player who plays in the position in question in an

**Table A1.7**

| Runs | |
| --- | --- |
| **Fig. A1.20:**<br>**Normal drill dosage** | **Two to three sets of four to eight runs** |
| Drill variation and progression options | |
| Intensity | To progress this drill using intensity, you can ask the player to work at a higher percent effort during the run phase. You could also use a hill with a gradient of 10–20 degrees to increase the intensity, but for this, runs of 20–30 m are sufficient. |
| Space | To progress this drill using space, you can adjust the distance covered in a run phase. Longer distance runs require more work than shorter distance runs at the same intensity. |
| Volume | To progress this drill using volume, the number of sets and repetitions can increase. |
| Movement | To progress this drill via the type of movement, if you feel appropriate, you can complete curved runs or runs with the player dribbling the ball. Just be sure you have a rationale for using this method of progression, e.g., to stimulate a healing adductor, as often adding more complex patterns of movement results in reduced running speed, which may have been your original goal. |
| Complexity | Not the best variable to progress runs. |
| Reaction | Not the best variable to progress runs. |

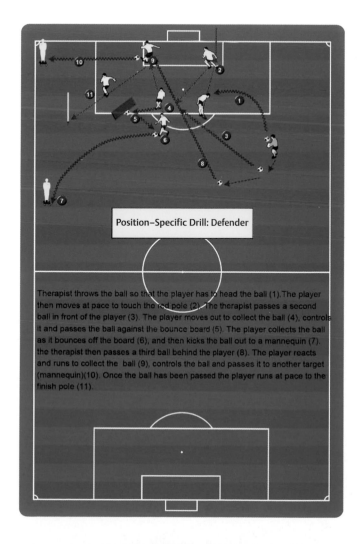

**Position–Specific Drill: Defender**

Therapist throws the ball so that the player has to head the ball (1). The player then moves at pace to touch the red pole (2). The therapist passes a second ball in front of the player (3). The player moves out to collect the ball (4), controls it and passes the ball against the bounce board (5). The player collects the ball as it bounces off the board (6), and then kicks the ball out to a mannequin (7). the therapist then passes a third ball behind the player (8). The player reacts and runs to collect the ball (9), controls the ball and passes it to another target (mannequin)(10). Once the ball has been passed the player runs at pace to the finish pole (11).

**Fig. A1.21**   Position-specific defender drill.

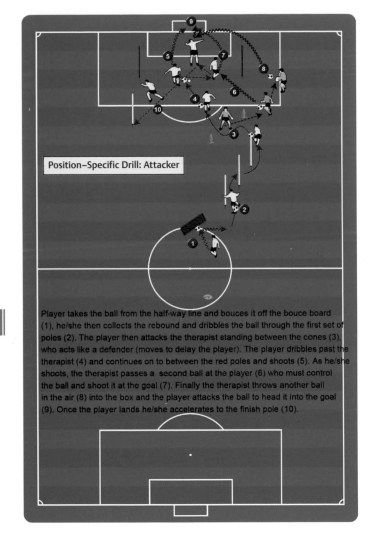

Player takes the ball from the half-way line and bouces it off the bouce board (1), he/she then collects the rebound and dribbles the ball through the first set of poles (2). The player then attacks the therapist standing between the cones (3), who acts like a defender (moves to delay the player). The player dribbles past the therapist (4) and continues on to between the red poles and shoots (5). As he/she shoots, the therapist passes a second ball at the player (6) who must control the ball and shoot it at the goal (7). Finally the therapist throws another ball in the air (8) into the box and the player attacks the ball to head it into the goal (9). Once the player lands he/she accelerates to the finish pole (10).

Position–Specific Drill: Attacker

**Fig. A1.22**   Position-specific attacking drill.

intense period of match play, you will see the sort of drill design you need. You can also combine specific pathology-based components in these drills. For example, if the injury were a thigh muscle injury, you would include a reactive sprint, or a shot toward a target. If the injury were an ankle sprain, you would include a jump-and-land component to challenge proprioception. Your imagination is your only limitation to the type of drill you design, but just remember if you want quality, then you need to design the drill to be challenging, but not so complex that the player cannot complete it with the quality you desire.

These drills will be intense and so you should not plan to do too many repetitions and you may want to include a good rest period between repetitions so you get quality movement. In a match, players do not run at high speed for long periods of time. Football is

an interval sport and so your rehab should reflect that.

### A1.2.16 Games

Games are an important part of a rehab progression, particularly when it is expected that there will be several sessions involved in the program (**Fig. A1.23**). Games allow recovery in terms of intensity, but still keep the player moving and focused; they can be used to achieve an outcome you want to achieve and they can also be very useful in building relationships with players because normally all players enjoy the challenge of a game. They can be designed to not challenge an injured area, by using the uninjured leg, or they can be designed to achieve a rehab goal, such as accurate strong passing. Three examples are included showing variations that will challenge the player to different levels. If you do not have the ability to kick the ball in a manner to

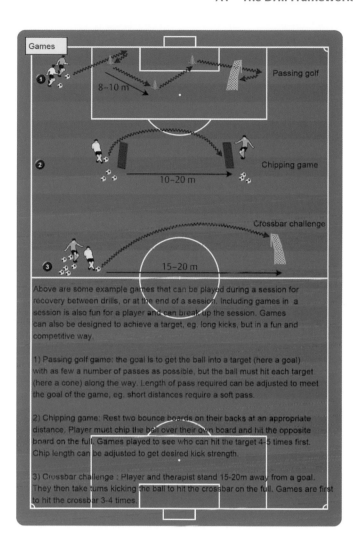

Fig. A1.23   Games.

compete against the player, then design games when the player needs to achieve a goal, such as pass the ball to knock over three cones on the goal with six passes. Professional football players play a game for a living. They love to compete, so use this desire to stimulate and develop the player in their rehab.

Once a player has passed through this progression, and performed the latter drills at high intensity and with quality, you can be confident that they can return to a training environment that recognizes that they will benefit from a controlled reintroduction to maximal training. How fast you progress a player through the drills and how you modify the drills along the way will depend on the diagnosis and the clinical presentation. In **Table A1.8**, two consecutive sessions are listed for a knee injury example for consideration. Highlighted in RED is where there has been a change between sessions, i.e., a progression of some form, so you can see what might be a logical

progression for a player. Again it is important to highlight that the degree of progression will reflect the pathology and in this case (a grade I medial collateral left knee ligament injury), you will see the progression is not overly aggressive but still that there is definite progress made.

## A1.3  Your Framework

As you develop your framework, you may choose to create a document such as that in **Fig. A1.24**. This document lists the various drills that are part of the framework that has been introduced earlier, in order of their progression. This document can then be used to plan your rehab. As a player completes a drill to a suitable level such that you are happy for them to progress, you can highlight or cross it off. When you plan your sessions, you can see where you need to go next and then by the

**Table A1.8**

Example of a progression of rehab session content between two early rehab sessions for a Grade I medial collateral knee ligament injury.

**Example progression of session content in consecutive sessions**

| Session 1 | Session 2 |
|---|---|
| **Warm-up:**<br>— Include passes with soft ball over 5 m<br>— Include basic proprioception drills | **Warm-up:**<br>— Include passes with normal ball over 10 m<br>— Include basic proprioceptive drills |
| **Multidirectional circuit without ball (no pass):**<br>— 1 × 60 s<br>— Rest 60 s | **Multidirectional circuit without ball (+ pass):**<br>— 1 × 60 s<br>— Rest 60 s |
| **Multidirectional circuit without ball (+ pass):**<br>— 1 × 60 s<br>— Rest 60 s | **Multidirectional circuit with ball:**<br>— 2 × 60 s<br>— Rest 60 s between sets. |
| **Multidirectional Circuit with ball:**<br>— 2 × 60 s<br>— Rest 60 s between sets. | **Passing:**<br>— Ten passes with left foot over 15 m |
| **Passing:**<br>— Ten passes with left foot over 5 m | **Four poles: predictable:**<br>— Level 1.5<br>— One set of eight touches<br>— One set of eight turns<br>— Rest 30 s between sets |
| **Four poles: predictable, touch poles:**<br>— Level 1<br>— Two sets of eight touches<br>— Rest 30 s between sets | **Four poles: unpredictable, touch poles:**<br>— Level 1<br>— Two sets of eight touches<br>— Rest 30 s between sets |
| **Four poles: predictable, touch poles:**<br>— Level 1<br>— Two sets of eight touches<br>— Rest 30 s between sets | **Passing:**<br>— Ten repetitions<br>— Chipping the ball over 10–15 m |
| **Game:**<br>— Passing golf game: only with noninjured legs<br>— Two to three minutes | **SAQ:**<br>— Levels 1.5–2<br>— Two sets of six different paths (10–15 s rest between each path)<br>— 1 min rest |
| **SAQ:**<br>— Level 1<br>— One set of six different paths (15–20 s rest between each path)<br>— One-minute rest | **Game:**<br>— Chipping game over 10 m<br>— Winner is first to four direct hits |
| **Passing:**<br>— Ten passes with left over 10 m | **Acceleration/deceleration:**<br>— Level 1<br>— Eight repetitions over 10 m |
| **Runs:**<br>— 4 × half pitch at 50% effort, walk second half of pitch for recovery | **Passing:**<br>— Ten passes with the left leg over 15 m |
| **Game:**<br>— Passing golf game to finish session.<br>— Two to three minutes | **Runs:**<br>— 4 × half pitch at 60% effort, slow jog second half of pitch for recovery |
| | **Game:**<br>— Chipping game over 15 m<br>— Winner is first to four hits on the full |

end of your progression you should have crossed off all the drills, and know you have "ticked all the boxes" of your framework. When all the drills have been ticked off, you can be confident you have implemented a thorough rehabilitation program and will hopefully NOT be "crossing your fingers" when the player returns to training.

| Player: *Player A* | Injury: *MCL Grade 1* | Date of injury: *01/01/15* | | | | |
|---|---|---|---|---|---|---|
| | | **Progression Levels** | | | | |
| **General Football Functional Movement** | | | | | | |
| Warm-Up | Jog, Static Stretch, MD Movts, Dynamic stretches, Light Ball Work | | | | | |
| MD Movt. without ball (pass only) | Level 1 (L1) | Level 2 (L2) | Level 2+ (L2+) | | | |
| MD Movt. with ball | Level 1 | Level 2 | Level 2+ | | | |
| Passing/Kicking | Soft Ball | Pass over 5-10m | Chipping the ball | Pass over 15m | Longer balls (200m+) | Shooting |
| | | | | | | |
| **Reaction, Agility, Accelerate/Decelerate** | | | | | | |
| Reactions: 4 poles with touch | L1 Predictable | L2 Predictable | L2+ Unpredictable | | | |
| Reactions: 4 poles with a turn | L1 Predictable | L2 Predictable | L2+ Unpredictable | | | |
| Speed, Agility, Quickness (SAQ) | L1 SAQ | L2 SAQ | | | | |
| Acceleration/Deceleration (A/D) | L1 A/D | L1 A/D + Turn (Combo) | L1 A/D (Combo) | L2+ A/D Combo | L2 SAQ + A/D Combo | L2+ SAQ + A/D Combo |
| | | | | | | |
| **Runs** | | | | | | |
| 1/2 Pitch (% effort) | 1/2 Pitch x4 (50%) | 1/2 Pitch x4 (60%) | 1/2 Pitch x6 (60%) | 1/2 Pitch x8 (60%) | 172 Pitch x6 (70%) | 1/2 Pitch x4 (80%) |
| | | | | | | |
| **Basic Strength/Power Exercises** | | | | | | |
| Lunge/Squat | L1 Squat/Lunge | L2 Squat/Lunge | Jump Squats | Split Jumps | Box Jumps | |
| | | | | | | |
| **Games** | | | | | | |
| Kicking | Glof (non injured leg) | Golf (injured leg) | Chipping Game | Kick at Targets | Crossbar Challenge | |
| | | | | | | |
| **Position Specific Drill** | | | | | | |
| Attacking | L1 | L2 | L2+ | | | |
| Defending | L1 | L2 | l2+ | | | |
| | | | | | | |
| **Variables to Consider for Sessions** | Sessions and Drill Volume and Duration | | | | | |
| | Drill Intensity (Level 1, 2, 3) | | | | | |
| | Drill Space (big vs small) | | | | | |
| | Reactions (predictable vs unpredictable) | | | | | |
| | Drill Complexity | | | | | |
| | Nature of Movement (type of movements) | | | | | |
| | Work-Rest (recovery between drills and sets) | | | | | |

A1

**Fig. A1.24** Functional framework drill progression document.

# Index